Gerontology:

An Annotated Bibliography

M. Leigh Rooke
Professor of Gerontology
School of Allied
Health Professions
Virginia Commonwealth University

C. Ray Wingrove
Chairman,
Department of
Sociology and Anthropology
University of Richmond

University Press
of America™

University Press of America™
division of
R.F. Publishing, Inc.
4710 Auth Place, S.E., Washington, D.C. 20023

Printed in the United States of America

ISBN: 0-8191-0232-6

PREFACE

This bibliography has been developed in response to inquiries not only from students but also from other individuals and organizations seeking reference materials in gerontology. Although the importance of periodical literature is acknowledged, such references have not been included. Only books, monographs and substantial papers are referenced in this bibliography, with the exception of some government publications. Major works are considered to be more accessable not only in libraries but also from publishing houses and for a longer life availability. The references included have been published between 1966 and early 1977, with exceptions made in some instances because of the continuing relevance of the publication or the paucity of materials on the topic.

ORGANIZATION OF THE BIBLIOGRAPHY

The materials are compiled in two major sections, namely, General References and Topical References. The Topical References include 33 subject categories, with cross references given when indicated for clarity. With few exceptions, individual topical categories have two components, one for books, major publications and monographs and a second for Federal Government publications. The latter group represents a sampling and is not to be construed as an exhaustive coverage. Additionally, the Federal publications are not annotated since the titles are found to be comprehensive descriptions of the contents.

Although journal articles have not been included in this bibliography, the final section of references is a list of selected journals and periodicals related specifically to aging. Knowledge of periodical literature is considered to be important to students of gerontology, since often the most current information available is found in these publications.

The compilers have incorporated a variety of references on the topics covered, recognizing that the knowledge base reflected in individual publications varies, and that the philosophies of the many authors reflect wide diversity. Even a cursory review of the contents under a number of topics demonstrates a dearth of writings in some areas, while in others there is essentially none. Perhaps this documented need for expanded information will stimulate both practitioners and academicians with the required competencies and knowledge to pursue studies and report findings on subjects for which materials available are sparse, and often limited to unsubstantiated value judgment.

ACKNOWLEDGEMENTS

Indebtedness in this undertaking is gratefully acknowledged to the individuals who have assisted in the search for gerontology references. To the libraries of the University of Richmond and Virginia Commonwealth University, to public and private agency personnel and to helpful colleagues, warm gratitude is given. Special appreciation is expressed to the University of Richmond for its financial support for preparation of the final manuscript, and to the secretary, Mrs. Miriam Rowe, who typed the drafts, struggled with illegibly penned revisions and maintained a viable sense of humor throughout the experience.

M. L. Rooke

C. Ray Wingrove

March, 1977

CONTENTS

GENERAL REFERENCES

Abernethy, J. B. Old Is Not a Four-Letter Word. Abingdon Press. Nashville, Tennesse. 1975.

A positive and optimistic view of old age as one stage in the life continuum.

Abrams, Margaret, and Robinson, Barry (Editors). National Leaders Speak Out on Options for Older Americans. The National Retired Teachers Association and the American Association of Retired Persons. Washington, D. C. 1971.

A compilation of excerpts from interviews with 46 prominent Americans.

Armour, Richard. Going Like Sixty: A Lighthearted Look at the Later Years. McGraw-Hill Book Company. New York, New York. 1975.

A retired author and humorist looks at aging and pokes gentle fun at the serious business of growing old.

Asquith, Glenn H. Living Creatively as an Older Adult. Herald Press. Scottsdale, Pennsylvania. 1975.

The author, who is retired, examines both the negative and positive aspects of aging from several perspectives, e.g., physical, social, financial, recreational, educational, psychological and spiritual.

Atchley, Robert C., and Seltzer, Mildred M. The Sociology of Aging: Selected Readings. Wadsworth Publishing Company. Belmont, California. 1976.

Selection of twenty readings comprise this book. Topics included are socialization, the family, economics, politics, and age and social stratification.

Balkema, John B. A General Bibliography on Aging. National Council on the Aging. Washington, D. C. 1972.

An annotated bibliography organized by categories that includes non-journal publications for the period 1967-1972.

Barry, John R., and Wingrove, C. Ray. *Let's Learn About Aging: A Book of Readings*. Schenkman Publishing Company, Inc. Cambridge, Massachusetts. 1977.

A comprehensive book of readings including selections in the following areas: demography; biological, psychological, and social aspects of aging; sex; retirement, death and dying; housing; social services; and treatment approaches.

Bart, Pauline, et al (Editors). *No Longer Young: The Older Woman in America*. Two Volumes. Institute of Gerontology. University of Michigan. Ann Arbor, Michigan. Vol. I, 1974. Vol. II, 1975.

I. *Work Group Reports*. Covers discussion and conclusions from 17 working groups in conferences held at the University.

II. *Occasional Paper in Gerontology, No. 11.* Covers conference plenary speeches.

Basic Concepts in Aging. Gerontology Center, Institute for the Study of Human Development. Pennsylvania State University. University Park, Pennsylvania. 1976.

Designed specifically for those having little academic background in gerontology, this manual provides general background knowledge of the aged and the aging process.

Baum, Daniel Joy. *The Final Plateau: The Betrayal of Our Older Citizens*. Burns & MacEacheon, Limited. Toronto, Ontario, Canada. 1974.

The author, a law school professor, has dealt with society's role in isolating and abandoning aging and aged persons in Canada. Evidence is given of the need to review and reassess retirement plans, pension systems, age oriented employment policies, and the social climate for growing old.

Beauvoir, Simone de. *The Coming of Age*. G. P. Putnam's Sons. New York, New York. 1972.

A readable, impressionist report and evaluation of society's treatment of the aged.

____________________. *Old Age*. Andre Deutsch, Ltd. and George Weidenfield and Nicolson, Ltd. London, England. 1972.

The author compares the old in present day society with the old in other times and places. Old age is considered in its totality, both biological and cultural.

Bell, Bill D. (Editor). Contemporary Social Gerontology. Charles C. Thomas. Springfield, Illinois. 1976.

A book of readings covering significant developments in the field of aging. Topics include: demography and ecology of aging; theories of aging; economics, housing and health, work, retirement and leisure; attitudes toward age and aging; family roles and social relations; morale, adjustment and life satisfaction; the minority elderly; the instutionalized elderly; and contemporary research strategies.

Bellak, L. The Best Years of Your Life: A Guide to the Art and Science of Aging. Atheneum Press. New York, New York. 1975.

Topical coverage includes not only the aging process, but also characteristics of the aged population in the United States and discusses places for retirement.

Benary-Isbert, Margot. These Vintage Years. Abingdon Press. Nashville, Tennessee. 1968.

At age 75 years, the author gives her views of old age, and she discusses life style modifications rather than dramatic change.

Benet, Sula. How to Live to Be 100: The Life Style of the People of the Caucasus. The Dial Press. New York, New York. 1975.

A study of the long-lived people of the Caucasus which includes nutritional information amounting to advice on how to attain longevity as well as the usual sociological data.

Bengtson, Vern L. Intergenerational Relations and Aging. The Ethel Percy Andrus Gerontology Center. University of Southern California. Los Angeles, California. 1975.

A bibliography.

Birren, James E. (Editor). Handbook of Aging and the Individual: Psychological and Biological Aspects. The University of Chicago Press. Chicago, Illinois. 1959.

Although an old publication, the fifth printing was made in 1971 and it still is considered helpful. Discusses the biological and psychological bases for aging changes. Good background in gerontology.

Birren, James E. (Editor-in-chief). The Handbooks of Aging Series. Van Nostrand Reinhold Company. New York, New York. 1977. (See topical listings for annotations.)

Vol. 1. Handbook of Aging and the Social Sciences.
Editor, Robert H. Binstock.

Vol. 2. Handbook of the Psychology of Aging.
Editors, James E. Birren, and K. Warner Schaie.

Vol. 3. Handbook of the Biology of Aging.
Editors, Caleb E. Finch and Leonard Hayflick.

Bier, William C. (Editor). Aging: Its Challenge to the Individual and to Society. Fordham University Press. New York, New York. 1974.

Number 8 in the Pastoral Psychology Series, this volume discusses a wide variety of topics related to aging, their ramifications and implications.

Bild, Bernice, R., and Havighurst, Robert J. Senior Citizens in Great Cities: The Case of Chicago. Part II, The Gerontologist, Volume 16, No. 1. The Gerontological Society. Washington, D. C. February, 1976.

A monograph prepared for the Chicago Mayor's Office for Senior Citizens, which reports the findings of a needs assessment follow up study to one made in 1972. The six subject groups included in the study were persons 60 years of age and older who were: homeowners, blacks, persons of Polish origin, residents of Rogers Park, persons living in residential hotels, and residents in public housing.

Blau, Zena Smith. Old Age in a Changing Society. Frank Watts. New York, New York. 1973.

An examination of problems associated with old age in contemporary society, with special attention to widowhood and retirement.

Boudreault, Marie-France, et al. Resources in Aging: To Live With Dignity. Institute of Gerontology. University of Michigan. Ann Arbor, Michigan. 1975.

Number five of a series of publications designed for practitioners and professionals. This one describes a program based on the concepts of milieu therapy in which a group of mentally and physically frail aged are drawn back into everyday living.

Boyd, Rosamonde, R., and Oakes, Charles G. (Editors). Foundations of Practical Gerontology, Revised Edition. University of South Carolina Press. Columbia, South Carolina. 1973.

Revision of papers presented at two institutes held at Converse College in 1967 with new chapters added. Includes sociology of aging, health and illness of the aged, psychological and psychiatric aspects of aging, economics of being old, and special programs and strategies for the aged.

Brantl, Virginia M., and Brown, Sister Marie Raymond (Editors). Readings in Gerontology. The C. V. Mosby Company. St. Louis, Missouri. 1973.

A collection of 12 articles ranging in subject from theories and research in aging to such specific areas as eating habits and suicide among older persons.

Burgess, E. W. (Editor). Aging in Western Societies. University of Chicago Press. Chicago, Illinois. 1960.

An early anthology of cross cultural comparisions of correlates of aging. This book has historical importance in gerontology.

Busse, Ewald W., and Pfeiffer, Eric (Editors). Behavior and Adaptation in Late Life. Little, Brown and Company. Boston, Massachusetts. 1969.

Seventeen authors cover a broad scope in the field of aging, giving clear concise summaries on many topics.

Butler, Robert N. Why Survive? Being Old In America. Harper & Row, Publishers, Inc. New York, New York. 1975.

Written by a physician, this book considers how a nation changes its attitudes toward the old and gives a strong indictment of social attitudes and treatment of the aged. Included is a discussion of problems confronting some of the aged, such as poverty, unemployment, housing, poor health.

Caldwell, Esther, and Hegner, Barbara R. Geriatrics: A Study of Maturity. Delmar Publishers. Albany, New York. 1975.

Although the title indicates that the book is limited to the medical specialty, geriatrics, it does in fact give an overview of aging, encompassing biological, psychological and social aging.

Carter, Ann P., et al. The Plus Years. Revised. Washington/Alaska Regional Medical Program. Safeco Insurance Companies. Seattle, Washington. 1974.

A compilation of articles on everyday aspects of growing older, which articles originally appeared in local newspapers throughout the state of Washington. They contain practical tips and suggestions for those who are aging.

Cober, Alan E. The Forgotten Society: 92 Drawings. Dover Publications. New York, New York. 1975.

Commentary combined with line drawings portray old as well as young institutionalized persons who have been forgotten or rejected by society.

Cobleigh, Ira U. Live Young as Long as You Live. Association Press. New York, New York. 1969.

Guidelines for a more productive, contented, and longer life.

Comfort, Alex. A Good Age. Crown Publishers. New York, New York. 1976.

An informative publication of a general nature, including demography, social and psychological considerations, health factors and prevalent disabilities. Has value for older persons and others interested in the subject.

Commitment to A Better Life: National Policy Concerns for Older Women. Federal Council on Aging. Washington, D. C. 1976.

A report focusing on national policy concerns for older women, with recommendations based upon hearings held in 1975 by the Federal Council on Aging.

Cowdry, E. V. Aging Better. Charles C. Thomas. Springfield, Illinois. 1972.

General survey of the field of aging, including physical, social, and emotional aspects; societal attitudes toward longevity.

Cowgill, Donald O., and Holmes, Lowell D. (Editors). *Aging and Modernization*. Appleton-Century-Crofts. New York, New York. 1972.

Cross-cultural study with wide-ranging coverage of subjects and societies. The contributing authors are sociologists, anthropologists, psychologists, and a social worker.

Current Literature on Aging. National Council on the Aging. Washington, D. C. Published quarterly.

An annotated bibliography updated quarterly which covers a number of topics.

Curtin, Sharon R. *Nobody Ever Died of Old Age*. Little, Brown and Company. Boston, Massachusetts. 1972.

An interesting and readable report by a nurse who wrote about her personal reactions to how society treats the aged.

Davies, David. *The Centenarians of the Andes*. Anchor Press/Doubleday. Garden City, New York. 1975.

The subject is the long-lived people of the Andes.

Davis, Richard H. *Television: A Therapeutic Tool for the Aged*. Ethel Percy Andrus Gerontology Center. University of Southern California. Los Angeles, California. 1975.

A brief "state of the art" summary of work in the area of television communication and the elderly; a narrative review of a three year study of the potential of television to enhance the lives of residents of communal facilities.

________________ (Editor). *Aging: Prospects and Issues*. Ethel Percy Andrus Gerontology Center. University of Southern California. Los Angeles, California. 1973.

A monograph composed of papers presented by authorities in the field of aging at a series of continuing education institutes. An overview of concerns related to aging.

Deeken, Alfons, S. J. *Growing Old and How to Cope With It*. J. Paulist Press. Paramus, New Jersey. 1972.

A positive approach to old age, dealing with problems and their solutions in relation to Christian principles and spiritual applications.

Degen, Charles. *Age Without Fear*. Exposition Press, Inc. Jericho, New York. 1972.

Written by a man in his nineties, the theme is about how to enjoy the later years of life by developing positive self-attitudes and concepts, and by acceptance of change with appropriate adaptation.

Deluca, L., et al. *Aging. An Annotated Guide to Governmental Publications*. Bibliography Series No. 3. University of Connecticut Library. Storrs, Connecticut. 1975.

A topical listing with brief description of material on aging available in government publications. Covers the period 1960-1974.

Estes, C. L., et al. *Developments and Trends in Aging: A Survey of Programs, Legislation, and Information Systems in a Sample of States*. California Commission on Aging. Sacramento, California. 1975.

Report of a project concerning current information on innovative trends and developments in aging, and their relevance to policy, legislation and programs. Emphasis is upon California.

Field, Minna. *Aging With Honor and Dignity*. Charles C. Thomas. Springfield, Illinois. 1968

This book discusses the economic, social, and familial areas of living in regard to their effect on the elderly.

____________. *Depth and Extent of the Geriatric Problem*. Charles C. Thomas. Springfield, Illinois. 1970.

The author includes a composite of problems and approaches to them, including the welfare of the elderly, difficulties encountered by older persons and their families, and the impact of the environment.

Gaffney, Sister Marie, and Wakin, Edward. Growing Old. Claretian Publications. Chicago, Illinois. 1972.

A survey of the physical, psychological, social and religious aspects of aging.

Geba, Bruno. Vitality Training for Older Adults: A Positive Approach to Growing Old. Random House. New York, New York. 1975.

A discussion of how the self-image of the aged might be brought in line with realities of the aging process.

General Bibliography on Aging, A. The National Council on the Aging, Inc. Washington, D. C. Revised periodically.

An annotated bibliography.

Golden Years...A Tarnished Myth, The. The Project FIND Report. National Council on the Aging. New York, New York. 1970.

A report on data compiled from twelve sections of the United States which documents and describes the conditions under which many older Americans live in later life.

Greenfeld, Josh, and Mazursky, Paul. Harry and Tonto. Saturday Review Press. E. P. Dutton and Company, New York, New York. 1974.

A charming story of an elderly man's travels with his cat, and about his independence and role identification.

Grey Sisters. Strategy for Tomorrow's Living: Extracts from Program, "Dynamics of Retirement," July 4-9, 1971. Grey Sisters Motherhouse. Pembroke, Ontario, Canada. 1971.

Report on a seminar on retirement, health and nutrition and spiritual accomodation to the aging process.

Gubrium, Jaber F. Time, Roles, and Self in Old Age. Behavioral Publications, Inc. New York, New York. 1975.

A resource book in gerontology dealing with such topics as: politics and the aged, the single elderly, the generation gap, and the effect of consistency in roles.

Hansen, Gary D., et al. Decade for Action in Gerontology and Geriatric Care; Education-Research-Services-Facilities: Long Range Plan 1966-1976. Mt. Angel College. Mt. Angel, Oregon. 1966.

Title self explanatory.

Hardy, R. E., and Cull, J. G. The Neglected Older Americans: Social and Rehabilitative Services. Charles C. Thomas. Springfield, Illinois. 1973.

A survey of common needs of the aged including health, financial support, religion, transportation and of some needed services.

Hendricks, Jon, and Hendricks, C. Davis. Aging in Mass Society: Myths and Realities. Winthrop Publishers. Cambridge, Massachusetts. 1977.

This book deals with the numerous dimensions and issues of aging, considering both the individual and society. The approach is both interdisciplinary and cross-cultural.

Hershey, Daniel. Lifespan and Factors Affecting It: Aging Theories in Gerontology. Charles C. Thomas. Springfield, Illinois. 1974.

A look at the theories of aging and related ideas.

Hoffman, Adeline M. The Daily Needs and Interests of Older People. Charles C. Thomas. Springfield, Illinois. 1970.

A good survey of the field of aging.

Huyck, Margaret Hellie. Growing Older. Prentice-Hall, Inc. Englewood Cliffs, New Jersey. 1974.

Exploration of the mental and physical changes, sexuality, work and leisure of older people; offers guidelines for living a long, satisfying life.

Ingleby, Betty, and Yorath, Margaret. Living With Old Age. Robert Hale Company. London, England. 1966.

Information for those who provide care to the elderly, including health and welfare services, living accomodations, and legal matters as they pertain to the aged population.

Isaacs, Bernard, et al. The Survival of the Unfittest. Blackwell Scientific Publications. Oxford, England. 1971.

Discussion of the challenge to society of having large numbers of ill,dependent people live into old age.

Jacobs, H. Lee, et al. Education for Aging: A Review of Literature. Eric Clearinghouse on Adult Education. Syracuse, New York. 1970.

A general coverage of the aging process in relation to problems and behavior patterns.

Jeffers, Frances C. (Editor). Proceedings of Seminars of the Duke University Council on Aging and Human Development: 1965-69. Center for the Study of Aging and Human Development. Duke University Medical Center. Durham, North Carolina. 1969.

Major addresses from seminars at Duke University including such topics as: geriatric research, methodology, health care, retirement, ecology, longevity.

Jonas, Doris, and Jonas, David. Young Till We Die. Coward, McCann and Geoghegan. New York, New York. 1973.

A discussion of attitudes toward the elderly and of roles of the aged in various societies; includes biological, psychological, and behavioral aspects of aging.

Jury, Mark, and Jury, Dan. Gramp. Grossman Publishers, New York, New York. 1976.

The story of a family that deals positively with the illness and death of an old member of the family. Profuse illustrations support the narrative in presenting a story that is both sad and beautiful.

Kalish, Richard A. (Editor). The Dependencies of Old People. Occasional Papers in Gerontology. Institute of Gerontology. University of Michigan. Ann Arbor, Michigan. 1969.

A collection of eight papers which examines the various kinds of dependency among the old.

Kalish, Richard A. Late Adulthood: Perspectives on Human Development. Brooks/Cole Publishing Company. Monterey, California. 1975.

A very readable book for the not-yet-old, giving basic facts and theoretical views regarding the late adult years. The book treats such topics as cognitive capacities, meaning of aging, mental functioning and the wide span of individual differences found among older people. Has a strong psychosocial emphasis.

Kastenbaum, Robert (Editor). Contributions to the Psychobiology of Aging. Springer Publishing Company, Inc. New York, New York. 1965.

A small volume which offers some of the thinking and research in the psychobiology of aging.

________________. New Thoughts on Old Age. Springer Publishing Company, Inc. New York, New York. 1964.

A survey of the field of aging, including characteristics of old age; includes social, psychological and therapeutic approaches to aging.

Kent, Donald P., et al (Editors). Research, Planning, and Action for the Elderly. Behavioral Publications. New York, New York. 1972.

A compilation of 31 papers which provides a comprehensive overview of current knowledge, identifies future trends in research, and suggests pertinent research methodologies and techniques. Informative text for theorists, researchers, and practitioners in the field of gerontology.

Kimmel, Douglas C. Adulthood and Aging: An Interdisciplinary, Developmental View. John Wiley and Sons. New York, New York. 1974.

Case illustrations of adults living varied and fulfilling lives in a study of human development from the middle years to old age and death. Emphasis is upon the interrelatedness of physiological, psychological and social aspects of aging.

Knopf, Olga. Successful Aging. Viking Press. New York, New York. 1975.

A discussion of the physical, social, and psychological aspects of aging by an 86 year old psychiatrist.

Leaf, Alexander, and Launois, John. Youth In Old Age. McGraw-Hill Book Company. New York, New York. 1975.

A very readable work on the centenarian populations of the Caucasus, U.S.S.R.; Hunza, West Pakistan; and Vilcabamba, Ecuador. Consideration is given to nutrition, exercise, genetics, work-rest ratios, mental attitudes and orientation as variables which might influence longevity.

Legislative Approaches to the Problems of the Elderly: A Handbook of Model State Statutes. Legal Research and Services for the Aged. National Council of Senior Citizens, Inc. Washington, D. C. March, 1971.

A catalogue of state statutes affecting the elderly; recommendations for a new, cohesive uniform legislative approach offered for consideration by the states.

Liang, Daniel S. Facts About Aging. Charles C. Thomas. Springfield, Illinois. 1973.

The layman is presented with the different changes which occur in the aging process.

Loether, Herman J. Problems of Aging. Second Edition. Dickenson Publishing Company. Encino, California. 1975.

A survey of sociological and psycho-social aspects and perspectives on problems of aging. A new chapter on widowhood added since the 1967 edition.

Lowenthal, Marjorie F., et al. Four Stages of Life. Jossey-Bass, Inc. San Francisco, California. 1975.

A report of the findings of in-depth study of four groups of men and women facing life transitions, including retirement; deals with stress, coping mechanisms, relationships, impact of sex roles, and other topics.

Maas, Henry S., and Kuypers, Joseph A. From Thirty to Seventy: A Forty-Year Longitudinal Study of Adult Life Styles and Personality. Jossey-Bass, Inc. San Francisco, California. 1974.

A report of findings from a longitudinal study of people assessed as young adults and then again when they were, on the average, seventy years old. These findings emphasize the increasing diversity among those growing old and the consequences of this diversity for planning and providing social services.

Maddox, George L. (Editor). *The Future of Aging and the Aged*. Southern Newspaper Publishers Association Foundation. Atlanta, Georgia. June, 1971.

A monograph summarizing a series of seminars; topics include theories of aging, economics, retirement, institutionalization, politics, research and training.

______________, and Karasik, Robin B. (Editors). *Planning Services for Older People: Translating National Objectives into Effective Programs*. Center for the Study of Aging and Human Development. Duke University Press. Durham, North Carolina. 1976.

This book reports and illustrates a strategy of policy research developed at the Duke University Center for the Study of Aging and Human Development and explores policies and programs of special relevance for older persons in the United States and the United Kingdom. The emergence of Area Agencies on Aging in the U.S. and decentralization of the British National Health Service are compared by professionals in each country as examples of organizational decentralization in terms of implications for policy formation and program implementation.

"Making the Knowledge Explosion Work for the Elderly," *Proceedings: 19th Annual Meeting of the Western Gerontological Society*, April 29-May 1, 1973. Los Angeles, California. 1974.

This report includes seven institutes covering such topics as law, nutrition, long term care, changing strategies for comprehensive services, religion, and national trends in public policy affecting the elderly.

Mandelbaum, Bernard. *Add Life to Your Years*. G. K. Hall. Boston, Massachusetts. 1974.

A book written for older persons, with major attention given to living fully in later life; published in large print for persons with vision problems.

Manney, James D., Jr. *Aging in American Society*. Institute of Gerontology. University of Michigan. Ann Arbor, Michigan. 1975.

A basic book dealing with concepts and processes of aging; reviews major public policy issues pertaining to the aged. Annotated references and appendix of other resources.

Match, Sondra K. (Editor). Health, Aging, Illness and Poverty. Senior Opportunities and Services. Technical Assistance Monograph No. 2. National Council on Aging. Washington, D. C. 1970.

An examination of hazards of old age, sickness, and poverty, and a look at the relief afforded by Medicare and Medicaid.

May, Siegmund H. The Crowning Years. J. B. Lippincott Company. Philadelphia, Pennsylvania. 1968.

The author, who is a physician, expresses his personal attitudes toward old age and describes how purposeful and gratifying aging can be.

McKinney, John C., and de Vyver, Frank T. (Editors). Aging and Social Policy. Appleton-Century-Crofts. New York, New York. 1966.

Topics cover retirement, employment and income maintenance, Federal and state programming, social services, housing, factors influencing health care of the aged, personality and aging, hospitals for the aged poor, and the social meaning of death.

McLeish, John A. B. The Ulyssean Adult. McGraw-Hill Book Company. New York, New York. 1976.

The author has utilized extensive resources in supporting his thesis that stereotyped old age is invalid. Documenting his stance on the vitality and creative pursuit in later life are the "Ulyssean Adults," all extraordinarily productive in old age.

McMorrow, Fred. Midolescence: The Dangerous Years. Strawberry Hill Publishing Company, Inc. New York, New York. 1974.

A report of personal observations made by the author of fourteen men and women representing various occupations and social life styles.

Merkin, Leon. The Old Age Story. Vantage Press, Inc. New York, New York. 1971.

This book is a guide and reference clarifying signs and symptoms of mental and physical illness and includes a section on retirement.

"Middle Years, The." American Journal of Nursing. Volume 75: 993-1024. June, 1975.

This is a special supplement in which nursing authorities explore emotional, physical, sexual and social changes, and point out ways to improve life style and enjoyment for a full life.

Mitchell, George. Yessir, I've Been Here a Long Time: The Faces and Words of Americans Who Have Lived a Century. E. P. Dutton and Company. New York, New York. 1975.

Using pictures and reports of memories and views of centenarians, the author demonstrates what they are like.

Moss, Bertram B., and Fraser, Kent. Caring for the Aged. Doubleday and Company, Inc. Garden City, New York. 1966.

Practical advice for those delivering services to the aged in the social, financial, medical, and psychological realms.

Moss, Gordon, and Moss, Walter (Editors). Growing Old. Pocket Books. New York, New York. 1975.

A book of essays and readings from artists and social scientists which depicts the life of the elderly in our youth oriented society and describes what the aged are doing to fight ageism in America.

Mow, Anna B. So Who's Afraid of Birthdays. J. B. Lippincott Company. Philadelphia, Pennsylvania. 1969.

This book is written by a seventy-five year old who found life more exciting and fulfilling as she aged. Her advice for meaningful aging has a strong religious orientation.

Munnichs, Joep M. A., and van den Heuvel, Wim J. A.(Editors). Dependency or Interdependency in Old Age. Martinus Nijhoff Publishers. The Hague, Netherlands. 1976.

This publication of the European Social Sciences Research Committee of the International Association of Gerontology presents findings of methodological studies concerning dependency, interdependency and autonomy.

Myth and Reality of Aging in America. The National Council on the Aging, Inc. Washington, D. C. 1975.

A 245 page report including charts, figures and detailed analysis of the Louis Harris survey to determine the public attitudes and perceptions of what it is like to be old in this country. Documents older Americans' views and attitudes about themselves.

Myth and Reality of Aging in America: A series of Monographs, The. National Council on the Aging, Inc. Washington, D. C. 1976.

A series of monographs analyzing specific areas of the Harris survey data. The monographs are as follows:

Setlow, Carolyn - An Interpretative Analysis of the Study
Tibbel, John - Mass Media
Havighurst, Robert J. - Education
Church, Frank - Federal Policy
Jackson, Maurice - Minorities
Lindsay, Inabel - Women
Abrams, Albert J. - State Policy
Meier, Elizabeth - Employment
Winston, Ellen - Service Providers

"Myths of Old Age Are the Myths of the Young: A Symposium, The." _Communication_. The Annenberg School of Communications. University of Pennsylvania. Philadelphia, Pennsylvania. Vol. 24, No. 4. Autumn, 1974.

An entire section of this issue (pp. 74-112) is devoted to discussion and analysis of some myths surrounding old age.

National Organizations With Programs in the Field of Aging. The National Council on the Aging, Inc. Washington, D. C. 1971.

A listing of 300 voluntary organizations with interest in the field of aging.

National Policy for Older Americans - Response to Their Special Needs, A. National Council of Senior Citizens. Washington, D. C. 1975.

A discussion of Federal programs for the aged including such topics as revenue sharing, employment programs, long term care, legal services, social security and nutrition.

"Old Age: The Individualist Triumphs." The Rotarian. December, 1974. Rotary International, 1600 Ridge Avenue. Evanston, Illinois. 1974.

An entire issue of the Rotarian devoted to the topic of the aged, includes papers by outstanding figures in the field of aging which take a positive look at aging.

Older Americans Act Project Management: Legal Duties and Responsibilities. The College of Law. Ohio State University. Columbus, Ohio. 1976.

This handbook intended for use by agencies and organizations offers an overview of the principal legal issues involved in operating a program and outlines potential problem areas. A wide variety of legal issues are covered including the nature of a Federal grant, HEW Regulations, Title VII Grants (illustrated by the Ohio Commission on Aging), Fair Labor Standards Act, etc.

"On Widowhood." Journal of Geriatric Psychiatry. No. 8. 1975.

This volume contains a series of papers presented at a symposium on widowhood.

Palmore, Erdman. The Honorable Elders: A Cross-cultural Analysis of Aging in Japan. Duke University Press. Durham, North Carolina. 1975.

An investigation of the status and social integration of the aged in Japan to be used as comparative data in studying aging in Western cultures.

____________ (Editor). Normal Aging I and II. Duke University Press. Durham, North Carolina. Vol. I, 1970; Vol. II, 1974.

Two volume report on the Duke Longitudinal Study.

I. For 1955-1969, this multidisciplinary study covers objectives and methods, health problems, intelligence, family and social areas,among other topics.

II. For 1970-1973, covers physical and mental aging, health care, social roles, self concepts, etc.

Percy, Charles H. Growing Old In the Country of the Young. McGraw-Hill Book Company. New York, New York. 1974.

A description of problems confronting the elderly; also suggests practical solutions.

Pfieffer, Eric. Functional Assessment: A Manual of Multidimensional Quantitative Evaluation of Functional State of Healthy and Impaired Adults. Older Americans Resources and Services Program. Duke University Center for the Study of Aging and Human Development. Duke University Medical Center. Durham, North Carolina. 1975.

This manual contains the rationale and specific techniques for assessing adults - especially aged adults - in four areas, viz., physical health, mental health, social resources, and economic resources.

______________ (Editor). Successful Aging: A Conference Report. Duke University Center for the Study of Aging and Human Development. Duke University Press. Durham, North Carolina. 1973.

Papers presented at the National Conference on "Successful Aging" held at Duke University in June, 1973. Conference papers focus on the paradox of successful aging, models of successful aging, and helping people to age successfully.

Prehoda, Robert W. Extended Youth: The Promise of Gerontology. G. P. Putnam's Sons. New York, New York. 1968.

An analysis of the major theories of the aging process associated with physical and mental decline.

Proceedings of the Annual Southern Conference on Gerontology. University of Florida Press. Gainesville, Florida. Annual publications.

Beginning in 1951 and continuing, the titles of the Proceedings of the Annual Southern Conference on Gerontology are as follows:

Vol. 1 Problems of America's Aging Population, edited by T. Lynn Smith, 1951.
Vol. 2 Living in the Later Years, edited by T. Lynn Smith, 1952.
Vol. 3 Health in the Later Years, edited by John M. Maclachlan, 1953.
Vol. 4 Economic Problems of Retirement, edited by George B. Hurff, 1954.
Vol. 5 Aging and Retirement, edited by Irving L. Webber, 1955.
Vol. 6 Aging: A Current Appraisal, edited by Irving L. Webber, 1956.
Vol. 7 Services for the Aging, edited by Irving L. Webber, 1957.
Vol. 8 Organized Religion and the Older Person, edited by Delton L. Scudder, 1958.
Vol. 9 Society and the Health of Older People, edited by Irving L. Webber, 1959.
Vol. 10 Aging: A Regional Appraisal, edited by Carter C. Osterbind, 1961.

Continued next page

Vol. 11 Aging in a Changing Society, edited by Ruth E. Albrecht (Xerographic "duplex" reproduction), 1962.
Vol. 12 Continuing Education in the Later Years, edited by J. C. Dixon, 1963.
Vol. 13 Social Change and Aging in the Twentieth Century, edited by Daniel E. Alleger, 1964.
Vol. 14 Maintaining High Level Wellness in Older Years, edited by Lois Knowles, 1965.
Vol. 15 Medical Care Under Social Security: Potentials and Problems, edited by Irving L. Webber, 1966.
Vol. 16 Income in Retirement: The Need and Society's Responsibility, edited by Carter C. Osterbind, 1967.
Vol. 17 Potentialities for Later Living, edited by O. Bruce Thomason, 1968.
Vol. 18 Feasible Planning for Social Change in the Field of Aging, edited by Carter C. Osterbind, 1969.
Vol. 19 Health Care Services for the Aged: Problems in Effective Delivery and Use, edited by Carter C. Osterbind, 1970.
Vol. 20 New Careers for Older People, edited by Carter C. Osterbind, 1971.
Vol. 21 Independent Living for Older People, edited by Carter C. Osterbind, 1972.
Vol. 22 Areawide Planning for Independent Living for Older People, edited by Carter C. Osterbind, 1973.
Vol. 23 Migration, Mobility, and Aging, edited by Carter C. Osterbind, 1974.
Vol. 24 Social Goals, Social Programs and the Aging, edited by Carter C. Osterbind, 1975.

Puner, Morton. *To the Good Long Life*. Universe Books. New York, New York. 1974.

A comprehensive, popularized version of what is known about growing old.

Quality of Life. American Medical Association. Publishing Sciences Group, Inc. Acton, Massachusetts. 1975.

A three volume publication of papers from three meetings of the National Congress on the Quality of Life. Covers the aging process throughout life.

Vol. 1 - Conception Through Adolescence.
Vol. 2 - Early and Mature Adulthood.
Vol. 3 - Opportunities and Strategies for Coping in Later Life.

Randel, William Pierce. *American Issues Forum.* National Council on the Aging. Washington, D. C. 1975. (A paperback kit).

Nine basic issues in American life are covered by the American Issues Forums from September, 1975 through May, 1976. NCOA has developed materials for the issues from an aging perspective.

Report on Conference on Aging and Long-Term Care. American Medical Association. Committee on Aging. Chicago, Illinois. 1965.

Subjects include: home care programs, homemaker services, retirement, nursing home care, adult education, community action, health insurance and rehabilitation.

Resources for the Aging: An Action Handbook. National Council on the Aging. New York, New York. 1969.

A comprehensive listing of private and public agencies, trusts and foundations which offer assistance to older people.

Riley, Matilda White, and Foner, Anne. *Aging and Society, Volume One: An Inventory of Research Findings.* Russell Sage Foundation. New York, New York. 1968.

Survey of the results of investigative studies in the field of aging; summarizes references by topic.

____________________, et al (Editors). *Aging and Society, Volume Two: Aging and the Professions.* Russell Sage Foundation. New York, New York. 1969.

Aging needs related to the contributions of a variety of professional disciplines.

____________________________________. *Aging and Society, Volume Three: Sociology of Age Stratification.* Russell Sage Foundation. New York, New York. 1972.

Delineation of arguments favoring use of age as a basis for social stratification.

Russ, Lavinia. *A High Old Time or How to Enjoy Being A Woman Over Sixty.* Sunday Review Press. New York, New York. 1972.

A practical and humorous guide to life for those over sixty written by one who has arrived there herself. The author deals with the joys as well as the hazards and frustrations of old age.

Saul, Shura. Aging: An Album of People Growing Old. John Wiley & Sons, Inc. New York, New York. 1974.

A collection of sensitive vignettes based upon interviews with aged persons. Illustrates attitudes of the elderly and their coping techniques in an urban community.

Schonfield, David, et al. A Basic Library of Books on Gerontology. University of Calgary. Alberta, Canada. 1969.

A basic resource for study of aging and the problems of the aged.

__________________, and Stewart, Robert. A Bibliography of Canadian Research in Gerontology, 1949-1969. University of Calgary. Alberta, Canada. 1970.

A comprehensive resource book on research by Canadians and designed as both a reference and as a tool "to increase interest in gerontological disciplines by showing how little and how much has been accomplished."

Schuckman, Terry. Aging is Not for Sissies. Westminster Press. Philadelphia, Pennsylvania. 1975.

A small volume that treats the condition of the aged in the United States, problems and attitudes, and the resulting status of the aged.

Schwartz, Arthur N., and Mensh, Ivan N. (Editors). Professional Obligations and Approaches to the Aged. Charles C. Thomas. Springfield, Illinois. 1974.

This is a book of papers prepared by 15 social scientists in the field of gerontology. The articles are oriented toward professionals working in the field of aging and offer information mation and suggestions to aid them in carrying out their responsibilities.

Scott, Frances Gillespie (Editor). Perspectives in Aging - Operational Focus. Oregon Center for Gerontology. Continuing Education Publication. Corvallis, Oregon. 1972.

Collection of readings which presents an overview of gerontology aimed toward the community college and lay audience.

Scott, Frances Gillespie. Perspectives in Aging - Research Focus. Oregon Center for Gerontology. Continuing Education Publication. Corvallis, Oregon. 1972.

Collection of readings which presents a multidisciplinary introduction to the study of gerontology.

Segerberg, Osborn, Jr. The Immortality Factor. E. P. Dutton and Company. New York, New York. 1974.

A discussion of the aging process presented in journalistic style but based upon both personal experience and scientific investigations.

Shanas, Ethel, and Sussman, Marvin B. (Editors). Family, Bureaucracy, and the Elderly. Duke University Press. Durham, North Carolina. 1977.

A collection of papers which considers how the aged cope with various bureaucratic structures, how family networks affect dealing with such structures, and how bureaucracies affect the relationships between old people and their families.

Shanks, Ann Zane. Old is What You Get. The Viking Press. New York, New York. 1976.

A series of dialogues about old age by old and young people.

Shock, Nathan. Current Publications in Gerontology and Geriatrics. Journal of Gerontology. Vol. 24. July, 1969.

A bibliography of materials classified by various aspects of aging.

______________. Trends in Gerontology. Second Edition. Stanford University Press. Stanford, California. 1957.

A historical review of gerontological developments in social, economic, psychologic, physiologic, and biologic areas.

Sinick, Daniel. Counseling Older Persons: Careers, Retirement, Dying. Human Sciences Press. New York, New York. 1977.

Primary concern is given to attitudes, motivation and obstacles related to career changes and retirement adjustment, as well as to income, housing, health, legal matters, and death including self-destructive behavior.

Smith, Bert Kruger. Aging in America. Beacon Press. Boston, Massachusetts. 1973.

A book dealing with the aged, their problems, and the programs designed to serve them. The way to develop a meaningful and enriched later life is considered in depth.

Smith, Elliott Dunlap. Handbook of Aging. Barnes and Noble. New York, New York. 1972.

A handbook for those growing old and for persons concerned about older persons. Deals with problems and their avoidance through preplanning.

"Sociological Aspects of Aging, The." Library Counselor. Vol. 20. April, 1965.

The entire issue constitutes an annotated bibliography on aging and includes the following subjects: economic insecurity, employment, retirement planning, social relationships, housing and recreation. Has historical value.

Spencer, Marian G., and Dorr, Caroline J.(Editors) Understanding Aging: A Multidisciplinary Approach. Appleton-Century-Crofts. New York, New York. 1974.

Emphasis is upon aging as a complex process and is designed for those who work with older persons. It is relevant for both education and research.

Steele, Harold C., and Crow, Charles B. How to Deal With Aging and the Elderly. The Strode Publishers. New York, New York. 1972.

Facts and interpretations from the field of gerontology written for professional and lay personnel in the social, religious, medical and nursing professions. Very simply written.

Sterne, Richard, S., et al. The Urban Elderly Poor. Lexington Books. Lexington, Massachusetts. 1974.

A study of the elderly poor in one Model Cities area with specific attention to, (1) behavior of elderly poor in an inner city and (2) effect of multiracial, inner-city environment upon the aged. Findings identify both racial and bureaucratic conflicts and offer implications for program planning and evaluation.

Stonecypher, D. D. Getting Older and Staying Younger. W. W. Norton and Company, Inc. New York, New York. 1974.

A book which argues that a normal old age, like a normal middle age or youth, can be healthy and vigorous even with physical handicaps as long as one's remaining physical and mental functions are exercised regularly. Practical advice, examples, and case histories are discussed.

Strugnell, Cecile. Adjustment to Widowhood and Some Related Problems: A Selective and Annotated Bibliography. Health Sciences Publishing Corporation. New York, New York. 1974.

A 201 page bibliography.

Swados, Harvey. Celebration. Simon and Schuster. New York, New York. 1975.

A novel written in the form of the diary of a 90 year old who finds himself torn by the pressures of opposing groups - one respecting his present status and the other agitating for his continued fight for radical ideas.

Taylor, Florence M. The Autumn Years: Insights and Reflections. Seabury Press. New York, New York. 1968.

Personal advice and philosophical views of a seventy-five year old.

Technical Bibliographies on Aging. The Ethel Percy Andrus Gerontology Center. University of Southern California. Los Angeles, California. 1975.

A series of topical bibliographies on aging which is comprised of the following:

Assessment and Therapy in Aging - Arthur N. Schwartz
Environmental Planning for the Elderly - Victor A Regnier, M. Arch.
Etiology of Mental Disorders in Aging - Arthur N. Schwartz
Intellectual Functioning and Aging - K. Warner Shail
Intergenerational Relations and Aging - Vern L. Bergston
Psychological Adjustment to Aging - Arthur N. Schwartz
Relations of Stress and Age - James E. Birren
Safety for the Elderly - Arnold M. Small
Sexuality and Aging - James E. Birren

Tibbitts, Clark, and Donahue, Wilma (Editors). Aging in Today's Society. Prentice-Hall, Inc. Englewood Cliffs, New Jersey. 1960.

An expanded revision of Aging in the Modern World first published in 1957 by the Fund for Adult Education.

Tiven, Marjorie Bloomberg. Older Americans: Special Handling Required. The National Council on the Aging. Washington, D. C. 1971. Reprinted 1975.

Brief survey of the status of older Americans written for a lay audience and covering health, income, food and nutrition, social services, transportation, institutional care and alternatives, and other areas of interest.

Tournier, Paul. Learn to Grow Old. Harper & Row, Publishers. New York, New York. 1971.

This book deals with a number of subjects of special importance to the aged, such as retirement, use of leisure time, loneliness, death and dying, suggests way to meet the challenges of growing old.

Troll, Lillian E. Early and Middle Adulthood. Brooks/Cole Publishing Company. Monterey, California. 1975.

The author relates theoretical knowledge to physiological, intellectual and psychological processes during the two life stages, and develops a life span perspective.

Twente, E. E. Never Too Old. Jossey-Bass Publishers. San Francisco, California. 1970.

Premised upon the concept that people are "never too old," the author points out directly and simply methods for helping elderly persons to achieve greater self awareness and richer lives in their communities.

Van Zonneveld, Robert J. Elderly People Living in Europe. Report on the International Association of Gerontology Colloquium, Paris, Bagnolet, April 1-3, 1971. International Center of Social Gerontology. Paris, France. 1972.

A general overview of Europe's aged population with special emphasis on employment and geriatrics.

Vedder, Clyde B. _Gerontology: A Book of Readings_. Second Printing. Charles C. Thomas. Springfield, Illinois. 1971.

Anthology covering a variety of topics.

________________ and Lefkowitz, Annette S. (Editors). _Problems of the Aged_. Charles C. Thomas. Springfield, Illinois. 1965.

Twenty-four contributors from a variety of disciplines write about problems found among the aged.

________________ (Editor). _Problems of the Middle-Aged_. Charles C. Thomas. Springfield, Illinois. 1965.

This book includes selections from the fields of medicine, psychology, sociology, and economics concerning the leading problems of the middle-aged.

Welford, A. T. (Editor). _Interdisciplinary Topics in Gerontology_. Buchdruckerai Pochon-Jent. A. G. Ben, Switzerland. 1969.

This book treats the different aspects of aging and aging change, and points out areas for needed research.

Woodruff, Diana S., and Birren, James E. (Editors). _Aging: Scientific Perspectives and Social Issues_. Ethel Percy Andrus Gerontology Center. University of Southern California. Los Angeles, California. 1975.

A comprehensive overview of the field of aging drawn from several scientific disciplines.

U. S. GOVERNMENT PUBLICATIONS

Action on Aging Legislation in 93rd Congress. Special Committee on Aging. United States Senate. Superintendent of Documents. U. S. Government Printing Office. Washington, D. C. February, 1975.

AOA Publications. Administration on Aging. U. S. Department of Health, Education, and Welfare. DHEW Publication No. (SRS) 73-20261. Superintendent of Documents. U. S. Government Printing Office. Washington, D. C. Updated periodically.

Amendments, Older Americans Act of 1965. Select Subcommittee on Education. Education and Labor Committee. Ninety-third Congress. First Session. U. S. House of Representatives. Superintendent of Documents. U. S. Government Printing Office. Washington, D. C. 1973.

Annual Report for the Year 1975. House Select Committee on Aging. Ninety-fourth Congress. U. S. Government Printing Office. Washington, D. C. 1976.

Annual Report to the President - 1975. Federal Council on the Aging. Department of Health, Education, and Welfare. Publication No. (OHD) 76-20955. Washington, D. C. 1975.

Commitment to a Better Life. Federal Council on the Aging. Washington, D. C. 1976.

Developments and Trends in State Programs and Services for the Elderly: A Survey of Activities at the State Governmental Level in the Field of Aging, 1972 and 1973. A report to the Special Committee on Aging. United States Senate. 93rd Congress, Second Session. U.S. Government Printing Office. Washington, D. C. November, 1974.

Developments and Trends in State Programs and Services for the Elderly. Report on a survey of activities at state government level in aging, 1974. Special Committee on Aging. U. S. Senate. Ninety-third Congress. Second Session. Superintendent of Documents. U. S. Government Printing Office. Washington, D. C. 1974.

Developments in Aging: 1974 and January-April, 1975. A report of the Special Committee on Aging. United States Senate. Ninety-fourth Congress. First Session. U. S. Government Printing Office. Washington, D. C. 1975.

Evaluation of Administration on Aging and Conduct of White House Conference on Aging. Ninety-second Congress. First Session. United States Senate. Special Committee on Aging. Superintendent of Documents. U. S. Government Printing Office. Washington, D. C. 1971.

Evaluation of Administration on Aging and Conduct of White House Conference on Aging. Special Committee on Aging and Subcommittee on Aging. Ninety-second Congress. Second Session. United States Senate. Superintendent of Documents. U. S. Government Printing Office. Washington, D. C. 1972.

Extramural Program of Research on Aging of the National Institute of Child Health and Human Development, Fiscal Year 1973, The. National Institute of Child Health and Human Development. U. S. Public Health Service. Bethesda, Maryland. 1974. Updated at regular intervals.

Facts About Older Americans, 1976. Administration on Aging. U. S. Department of Health, Education and Welfare. Publication No. (OHD) 75-20006. Superintendent of Documents. U. S. Government Printing Office. Washington, D. C. 1976. Updated annually.

Foreign Programs for Elderly. Office of International Affairs. U.S. Department of Housing and Urban Development. Washington, D. C. 1973.

Golden Years, Tarnished Myth: Project FIND Report. National Council on the Aging. Economic Opportunity Office. Executive Office of the President. Superintendent of Documents. U. S. Government Printing Office. Washington, D. C. 1970.

Government's Response to The Elderly. Introduction to the Administration on Aging. Hearing Before the Select Committee on Aging. House of Representatives. Superintendent of Documents. U. S. Government Printing Office. Washington, D. C. 1975.

Hearings to Amend Older Americans Act of 1965. Select Subcommittee on Education. Education and Labor Committee. Ninety-second Congress. First Session. U. S. House of Representatives. Superintendent of Documents. U. S. Government Printing Office. Washington, D. C. 1972.

Interrelationship of Benefit Programs for the Elderly, The. The Federal Council on the Aging. U. S. Department of Health, Education and Welfare. National Clearing House on the Aging. Washington, D. C. 1976.

Introduction to the Administration on Aging, September 24, 1975. Presentation of Arthur S. Flemming, U. S. Commissioner on Aging. Hearings Before the House Select Committee on Aging. Ninety-fourth Congress. Superintendent of Documents. U. S. Government Printing Office. Washington, D. C. 1975.

Legislative History of Older Americans Comprehensive Services Amendments of 1972. Subcommittee on Aging of Committee on Labor and Public Welfare and Special Committee on Aging. Labor and Public Welfare Committee. Ninety-second Congress. Second Session. U. S. Senate. Superintendent of Documents. U. S. Government Printing Office. Washington, D. C. 1972.

Let's End Isolation. U. S. Department of Health, Education and Welfare. Social and Rehabilitation Service. Administration on Aging. AOA Publication No. 129. Superintendent of Documents. U. S. Government Printing Office. Washington, D. C. June, 1971.

Message From the President of the United States; Transmitting Recommendations for Action on Behalf of the Older Americans. Superintendent of Documents. U. S. Government Printing Office. Washington, D. C. 1972.

National Clearinghouse on Aging, November 6, 1975. Presentation by Donald F. Reilly, Deputy Commissioner on Aging, and Clark Tibbitts, Director of the National Clearinghouse on Aging. Hearings before the House Select Committee on Aging. Ninety-fourth Congress. Superintendent of Documents. U. S. Government Printing Office. Washington, D. C. 1975.

National Institute of Aging: Hearing. Subcommittee on Public Health and Environment, Interstate and Foreign Commerce Committee. Ninety-second Congress. First Session. U. S. House of Representatives. Superintendent of Documents. U. S. Government Printing Office. Washington, D. C. 1972.

National Policy Concerns for Older Women: Commitment to A Better Life. Federal Council on the Aging. U. S. Department of Health, Education and Welfare. Publication No. (OHD) 76-20956. Washington, D. C. 1975.

Needs of Veterans and Widows 72 Years of Age or Older. Veterans Affairs Committee. U. S. Senate. Ninety-fourth Congress. First Session. Veterans Administration. Washington, D. C. 1975.

Older Americans, A National Resource. Administration on Aging. U. S. Department of Health, Education and Welfare. DHEW Publication No. (OHD/AOA) 74-20810. Superintendent of Documents. U. S. Government Printing Office. Washington, D. C. 1974.

Older Americans Act and the Rural Elderly, The. Hearing before the Special Committee on Aging. U. S. Senate. Ninety-fourth Congress. First Session. U. S. Government Printing Office. Washington, D. C. April 28, 1975.

Older Americans Act of 1965: 1973 Revision. Public Law 93-29. Ninety-third Congress. S. 50. Older Americans Comprehensive Services Amendments of 1973. Superintendent of Documents. U. S. Government Printing Office. Washington, D. C. May, 1973.

Older Americans Act of 1965, As Amended and Related Acts. Administration on Aging. Office of Human Development. U. S. Department of Health, Education and Welfare. Publication No. (OHD) 76-20170. Superintendent of Documents. U. S. Government Printing Office. Washington, D. C. 1976.

Older Americans Act Amendments of 1972. Subcommittee on Aging. Labor and Public Welfare Committee. Ninety-second Congress. Second Session. U. S. Senate. Superintendent of Documents. U. S. Government Printing Office. Washington, D. C. 1972.

Older Americans Act Amendments, 1973. Subcommittee on Aging. Labor and Public Welfare Committee. Ninety-third Congress. First Session. U. S. Senate. Superintendent of Documents. U. S. Government Printing Office. Washington, D. C. 1973.

Older Americans Comprehensive Services Amendments of 1973. Special Committee on Aging. Ninety-third Congress. First Session. U. S. Senate. Superintendent of Documents. U. S. Government Printing Office. Washington, D. C. 1973.

Oversight Hearings on Older Americans. Select Subcommittee on Education and Labor Committee. Ninety-third Congress. First and Second Sessions. U. S. House of Representatives. Superintendent of Documents. U. S. Government Printing Office. Washington, D. C. December 3, 1973, and February 13, 1974.

Post-White House Conference on Aging Reports, 1973: Towards A New Attitude on Aging. Special Committee on Aging. Subcommittee on Aging. Committee on Labor and Public Welfare. U. S. Senate. Superintendent of Documents. U. S. Government Printing Office. Washington, D. C. 1973.

Pre-White House Conference on Aging: Summary of Development and Data. Special Committee on Aging. Ninety-second Congress. First Session. U. S. Senate. Superintendent of Documents. U. S. Government Printing Office. Washington, D. C. 1971.

Problems of the Aging Hearings. Subcommittee on Aging. Government Operations Committee. Ninety-second Congress. First Session. U. S. House of Representatives. Superintendent of Documents. U. S. Government Printing Office. Washington, D. C. 1972.

Problems of Aging. Subcommittee on Aging. Government Operations Committee. Ninety-Second Congress. Second Session. U. S. Senate. Superintendent of Documents. U. S. Government Printing Office. Washington, D. C. 1972.

Proposed Fiscal 1976 Budget, The: What It Means for Older Americans. A Staff Report, Special Committee on Aging. United States Senate. Ninety-fourth Congress. Superintendent of Documents. U. S. Government Printing Office. Washington, D. C. 1975.

Publications List. Special Committee on Aging. United States Senate. Eighty-seventh-Ninety-fourth Congresses. Superintendent of Documents. U. S. Government Printing Office. Washington, D. C. 1976.

Reports of the Special Concerns Sessions. White House Conference on Aging. U. S. Government Printing Office. Washington, D. C. 1972. The Recommended for Action Series.

Vol. 1 - Aging and Aged Blacks.
Vol. 2 - Aging and Blindness: Physical and Vocational Rehabilitation of Older People; and Reports on Aging and Deafness.
Vol. 3 - Asian American Elderly.
Vol. 4 - Elderly Indians.
Vol. 5 - Long-term Care for Older People; Mental Health Care Strategies and Aging; Homemaker-Home Health Aide Services.
Vol. 6 - Older Family; The Religious Community and the Aging; The Elderly Consumer; Legal Aid and the Urban Aged.

Research in Aging, 1972. Subcommittee on Aging. Labor and Public Welfare Committee. Ninety-second Congress. Second Session. U.S. Senate. Superintendent of Documents. U. S.Government Printing Office. Washington, D. C. 1972.

Research on Aging Act. Subcommittee on Aging. Labor and Public Welfare Committee. Ninety-third Congress. First Session. U. S. Senate Superintendent of Documents. U.S. Government Printing Office. Washington, D. C. 1973.

Review of Public Policy by the National Council on the Aging. Hearing before the Select Committee on Aging. House of Representatives. Ninety-Fourth Congress. First Session. Superintendent of Documents. U. S. Government Printing Office. Washington, D. C. 1975.

Rich, Thomas A., and Gilmore, Alden S. Basic Concepts of Aging: Programmed Manual. Administration on Aging. U. S. Department of Health, Education and Welfare. DHEW Publication No. (SRS) 72-20274. Superintendent of Documents. U. S. Government Printing Office. Washington, D. C. 1972.

Society's Responsibilities to the Elderly. Presentation by Dr. Robert Butler, Director of National Institute of Aging. Hearings before the House Select Committee on Aging, November 11, 1975. Ninety-Fourth Congress. Superintendent of Documents. U. S. Government Printing Office. Washington, D. C. 1975.

State of Aging, The. Hearing before the House Select Committee on Aging, June 9, 1975. Superintendent of Documents. U. S. Government Printing Office. Washington, D. C. 1975.

To Find the Way to Opportunities and Services for Older Americans. U. S. Administration on Aging. Washington, D. C. 1975.

Toward a Brighter Future for the Elderly. U. S. President's Task Force on the Aging. Superintendent of Documents. U. S. Government Printing Office. Washington, D. C. 1970.

Toward a National Policy on Aging. White House Conference on Aging, November 28-December 2, 1971. Superintendent of Documents. U. S. Government Printing Office. Washington, D. C. 1973.

White House Conference on Aging, 1971: Background and Issues. Fourteen Background Papers. U. S. Department of Health, Education and Welfare. Administration on Aging. Washington, D. C. 1971.

"Education"
"Employment and Retirement"
"Facilities, Programs and Services"
"Government and Non-government Organization"
"Housing"
"Income"
"Nutrition"
"Physical and Mental Health"
"Planning"
"Research and Demonstration"
"Retirement Roles and Activities"
"Spiritual Well-Being"
"Training"
"Transportation"

White House Conference on Aging, 1971. Ninety-Second Congress. First Session. U. S. Senate. Superintendent of Documents. U. S. Government Printing Office. Washington, D. C. 1971.

Words On Aging: A Bibliography of Selected Annotated References. Administration on Aging. U. S. Department of Health, Education and Welfare. U. S. Government Printing Office. Washington, D. C. 1970.

More Words on Aging: Supplement, 1971.

References compiled by subjects for journal articles (1963-1967) and books (1900-1967). The supplement covers the period 1968-1970.

Working With Older People: A Guide to Practice. Four Volumes. U. S. Department of Health, Education and Welfare. U. S. Public Health Service. Public Health Service Publication No. 1459. Superintendent of Documents. U. S. Government Printing Office. Washington, D. C. 1969-1970.

Volume I - The Practitioner and the Elderly.
Volume II - Biological, Psychological and Sociological Aspects of Aging.
Volume III - The Aging Person: Needs and Services.
Volume IV - Clinical Aspects of Aging.

TOPICAL REFERENCES

AGING, BIOLOGICAL AND PHYSIOLOGICAL

Andrew, Warren. The Anatomy of Aging in Man and Animals. Grune and Stratton. New York, New York. 1971.

An analysis is made of structural aging, covering the gamut from protozoa to man.

Bakerman, Seymour (Editor). Aging Life Processes. Charles C. Thomas. Springfield, Illinois. 1969.

Biochemical knowledge is related to the process of aging.

Balazs, Andras, et al. Reproduction and Aging. MSS Information Corporation. New York, New York. 1973.

A discussion of the effects of reproduction on aging, including fertility and aging, ovarian and testicular function and aging, and the effect of castration on life span.

Bertolini, Alberto M. Gerontologic Metabolism. Charles C. Thomas. Springfield, Illinois. 1969.

A summary of the literature prior to 1969 on cross-cultural studies in the biochemistry of senescence. Translated from the Italian.

Brody, Harold, et al (Editors). Aging - Vol. 1: Clinical, Morphologic, and Neurochemical Aspects in the Aging Central Nervous System. Raven Press. New York, New York. 1975.

A compilation of studies from several disciplines showing the relationship of changes in the central nervous system to aging. Both current knowledge and identification of knowledge gaps are included.

Burch, Philip R. J. An Inquiry Concerning Growth, Disease and Aging. Oliver and Boyd. Edinburgh, Scotland. 1968.

An exploration into the breakdown of the homeostatic system controlling tissue growth and its relationship to the appearance of diseases and conditions of aging.

Burnet, Sir Macfarlane. *Intrinsic Mutagenesis: A Genetic Approach to Aging*. John Wiley and Sons, Inc. New York, New York. 1974.

A technical book which challenges the theory that the lifespan of a mammal is genetically determined and the process results in accumulated genetic error and mutations.

____________. *The Biology of Aging*. Oxford University Press. New York, New York. 1975.

This is a more simplified, shorter treatment of the author's *Intrinsic Mutagenesis: A Genetic Approach to Aging*, which was published in 1974.

Comfort, Alex. *Ageing: The Biology of Senescence*. Revised Edition. Holt, Rinehart and Winston, Inc. New York, New York. 1964.

A study of the biology of aging, why it occurs, whether it is controllable, and how control may be achieved.

Cristofalo, Vincent J., et al (Editors). *Explorations in Aging*. Plenum Publishing Corporation. New York, New York. 1975.

A compilation of selected research studies related to three major biological areas pertaining to aging: cell division, hormonal regulatory mechanisms, and the cardiovascular system and functions.

____________________, and Holečková, Emma (Editors). *Cell Impairment in Aging and Development*. Plenum Publishing Corporation. New York, New York. 1975.

The proceedings of an international symposium held in Czechoslovakia on "Impairment of Cellular Functions During Aging and Development in Vivo and in Vitro."

Curtis, Howard J. *Biological Mechanisms of Aging*. Charles C. Thomas. Springfield, Illinois. 1966.

An examination of biological theories of aging within contemporary conceptual frameworks.

Cutler, R. G. (Editor). Cellular Ageing: Concepts and Mechanisms, Parts I and II. Volumes 9 and 10, Interdisciplinary Topics in Gerontology. S. Karger. New York, New York. 1976.

An authoritative, technical treatment of cellular aging, including adaptations and differentiation, genetic factors, among others, in both man and other animals.

Dirkin, Johan Maurits (Editor). Functional Age of Industrial Workers. Institute for Preventive Medicine. TNO Wolters-Noordhoff. Graningen, Netherlands. 1972.

Report of a survey of capacities of the aging and delineation of the method for assessing functional age.

Edge, J. R., et al. The Aging Lung: Normal Function. MSS Information Corporation. New York, New York. 1973.

Detailed description of the aging lung, including cellular, molecular, and physiological components.

Everitt, Arthur V., and Burgess, John A. (Editors). Hypothalmus, Pituitary and Aging. Charles C. Thomas. Springfield, Illinois. 1976.

An authoritative reference on the subject of endocrines and their age relationships. One section is devoted primarily to functional age changes; other chapters consider endocrine effects upon skeletal, cardiovascular and other systems. Old concepts are reviewed and new ones included.

Finch, Caleb Ellicott. Cellular Activities During Aging in Mammals. MSS Information Corporation. New York, New York. 1972.

A comprehensive biological cellular review of aging in mammals.

__________________, and Hayflick, Leonard. Handbook of the Biology of Aging. Van Nostrand Reinhold Company. New York, New York. 1977.

Volume 3, Handbooks of Aging Series, covers aging from the comparative biological and evolutionary points of view, and examines age change at many levels. Both humans and other mammals are considered in the biological aging process.

Gaitz, Charles M. (Editor). Aging and the Brain. Plenum Press. New York, New York. 1972.

Proceedings of the fifth annual symposium held at the Texas Research Institute of Mental Sciences in 1971. Papers presented covered a number of neurological research studies and findings.

Gey, K. F., et al Structure and Chemistry of the Aging Heart. MSS Information Corporation. New York, New York. 1974.

A discussion of biochemistry, heart valves, amyloidosis, vascularity, and ultrastructure of the aging heart.

Gitman, Leo. Endocrines and Aging. Charles C. Thomas. Springfield, Illinois. 1967.

Report of a symposium presented before the 17th annual meeting of the Gerontological Society.

Goldman, Ralph, and Rockstein, Morris (Editors). The Physiology and Pathology of Aging. Academic Press, Inc. New York, New York. 1975.

The proceedings of a symposium on human aging held in Miami, Florida, in 1975. A variety of normal as well as pathological physiological processes of aging are discussed.

Gutmann, Ernest, and Hanzlikova, V. Age Changes in the Neuromuscular System. Scientechnica Publishers, Ltd. Bristol, England. 1972.

Title self explanatory.

Hall, David A. Elastolysis and Aging. Charles C. Thomas. Springfield, Illinois. 1964.

Consideration of the possible effects of enzymes in the aging of elastic tissue.

____________. The Aging of Connective Tissue. Academic Press. New York, New York. 1976.

The author, a biochemical gerontologist, advances new theories on the relationship between structure and function and the development and aging of humans. Recent research is reviewed.

Imaizumi, Tadahoshi. Growth, Maturation and Aging. Kugayama Press. Tokyo, Japan. 1976.

A small book written in clear English which deals with nutrition, theories of aging as well as cause and effect relationships in growth, maturation and aging.

Kohn, Robert R. Principles of Mammalian Aging. Prentice-Hall, Inc. Englewood Cliffs, New Jersey. 1971.

A book concerned with the aging process at different levels of organization; the cause-and-effect sequences, and the basic chemistry and structure of living systems.

Krohn, Peter L. (Editor). Topics in the Biology of Aging: A Symposium Held at the Salk Institute for Biological Studies. Interscience Publishers, Inc. New York, New York. 1966.

A critical look at research in the biology of aging.

Milne, Lorus J., and Milne, Margery. The Ages of Life. Harcourt, Brace and World. New York, New York. 1968.

The authors trace the pattern of growth in all living things, discuss findings on growth and aging, and the application of scientific knowledge to the extension of useful human life.

Montagna, William (Editor). Aging: Proceedings of the Symposium Held at the University of Oregon Medical School, 1964. Pergamon Press. New York, New York. 1965.

Characteristics of and processes involved in aging skin.

Nanda, B. S., et al. Aging Pigment, I: Current Research. MSS Information Corporation. New York, New York. 1974.

A description of the distribution and ultrastructure of aging pigments and the mechanisms which influence the rate of accumulation.

Norris, A. H., et al. *The Central Nervous System and Aging*. MSS Information Corporation. New York, New York. 1973.

An examination of research on age related changes in the central nervous system covering such topics as: impulse conduction velocity and reflexes, metabolism and cellular regulation, changes in neurotransmitter activities, electroencephalography, and cerebral blood flow in the aged.

Ordy, J. M., and Brizzee, K. R. (Editors). *Neurobiology of Aging*. Plenum Publishing Corporation. New York, New York. 1975.

This is an interdisciplinary life-span approach to study of the human brain, and deals with selected research and research trends in the area of functional and structural changes caused by aging.

Palmore, Erdman B., and Jeffers, Frances C. *Prediction of Life Span*. Lexington Books, D. C. Heath and Company. Lexington, Massachusetts. 1971.

A summary of relevant findings pertinent to longevity of humans.

Proceedings of Seminars, 1965-1969. Council on Aging and Human Development. Duke University. Durham, North Carolina. 1969.

A report of geriatric research, e.g., methodology, psychophysiological aspects, health care, ecology, retirement, mortality, and longevity.

Robert, L., and Robert, Barbara (Editors). *Aging of Connective Tissues - Skin*. S. Karger. New York, New York. 1973.

The proceedings of the Eleventh International Colloquium of Dermo-Chemistry on Aging of Skin held in Paris in 1972. The papers cover a number of topics related to subject.

Robertson, O. H., et al. *Endocrines and Ageing*. MSS Information Corporation. New York, New York. 1972.

A collection of articles on the study of the aging process presenting evidence of changes in the endocrine system of aging mammals.

Rockstein, Morris (Editor). Development and Aging in the Nervous System. Academic Press. New York, New York. 1973.

A collection of papers by research scientists which covers a wide range of topics "from embryological development through senility."

__________________, and Baker, George T., III (Editors). Molecular Genetic Mechanisms in Development and Aging. Academic Press. New York, New York. 1972.

A report of on-going research in the areas of nucleic acids and protein metabolism related to human development and aging.

__________________, et al (Editors). Theoretical Aspects of Aging. Academic Press. New York, New York. 1974.

The fourth volume in the series reporting symposium proceedings on cellular aging by the Department of Physiology/Biophysics and of Microbiology of the School of Medicine, University of Miami. An authoritative review of theories of aging, related influences and research findings.

Rose, Charles L., and Bell, Benjamin. Predicting Longevity: Methodology and Critique. D. C. Heath and Company. Lexington, Massachusetts. 1971.

Critical, systematic review of the research methods and findings on longevity up to 1970; descriptive analysis of sophisticated experimental processes adapted to the study of longevity.

Rosenfeld, Albert. Prolongevity. Alfred A. Knopf. New York, New York. 1976.

The author, a scientific journalist, gives a simple presentation on biology of aging, including current concepts and research taking place.

Sensory Deprivation and the Elderly. Gerontology Center. Institute for the Study of Human Development. Pennsylvania State University. University Park, Pennsylvania. 1976.

The major goal of this training program is to instill empathic understanding of those suffering sensory loss in order to improve social interactions between service providers and the elderly.

Shock, Nathan W. (Editor). *Perspectives in Experimental Gerontology*. Charles C. Thomas. Springfield, Illinois. 1966.

Biological and physiological aspects of aging; an examination of theories of aging and of the future in aging research.

Stracher, Alfred (Editor). *Aging in Muscles*. (Vol. 4, *Aging* Series). Raven Press. New York, New York. (In press).

A report on studies and the status of research concerning the relationship of aging to changes in muscles.

Talland, George A. (Editor). *Human Aging and Behavior: Recent Advances in Research and Theory*. Academic Press, Inc. New York, New York. 1968.

The thesis is to relate age associated changes in performance to parallel biological function changes in the aging organism.

Terry, Robert D., and Gershon, Samuel (Editors). *Aging*. (Series on Gerontology). Raven Press. New York, New York.

Vol. 1. *Clinical Morphologic and Neurochemical Aspects in the Aging Central Nervous System*. Edited by Harold Brody, Denham Harman, and J. Merk Ordy. 1975.

Vol. 2. *Genesis and Treatment of Psychologic Disorders in the Elderly*. Edited by Samuel Gershon and Allen Raskin. 1975.

Vol. 3. *Neurobiology of Aging*. Edited by Robert D. Terry and Samuel Gershon. 1976.

Vol. 4. *Aging in Muscles.* Edited by Alfred Stracher. (In press).

____________________. *Neurobiology of Aging*. (Vol. 3, Series *Aging*). Raven Press. New York, New York. 1976.

A comprehensive examination of topics of significance in the aging nervous system, covering physiology, morphology and neuroanatomy, immunology and endocrinology and neurochemistry.

Thorbecke, Jeanette (Editor). *The Biology of Aging and Development.* Plenum Publishing Corporation. New York, New York. 1975.

An interdisciplinary reference book on current research pertaining to development and aging by immunologists, cell biologists, pathologists, among others. Some sociological aspects of aging also are given attention.

Timiras, P. S. *Developmental Physiology and Aging.* The Macmillan Company. New York, New York. 1972.

A resource book dealing with physiological changes that occur during the life span.

Van Keep, P. A., and Ch. Lauritzen (Editors). *Ageing and Estrogens.* Frontiers of Hormone Research, Vol. 2. S. Karger. New York, New York. 1973.

An authoritative treatment of biological and physiological changes in the aging woman, psychic effects, therapy.

Walford, R. L., et al. *The Relation of Aging to Immunity.* MSS Information Corporation. New York, New York. 1973.

Papers presented deal with immunological effects of aging in relation to disease states, malignancies, autoimmunity and immunologic tolerance.

Weale, Robert A. *The Aging Eye.* Harper and Row Publishers, Inc. New York, New York. 1963.

Broad survey of what is known about age related changes in the eye. Despite the age of the book, it is one of the few available references on this topic.

Welford, A. T., and Birren, James E. (Editors). *Behavior, Aging, and the Nervous System: Biological Determinants of Speed of Behavior and Its Changes With Age.* Charles C. Thomas. Springfield, Illinois. 1965.

Title self explanatory.

Winter, Ruth. *Ageless Aging.* Crown Publishers. New York, New York. 1973.

Emphasis is upon biological and physiological changes among other topics; explores hormonal changes related to the aging process.

Wright, E. A., et al. Brain Structure and Aging. MSS Information Corporation. New York, New York. 1974.

A summary of up-to-date, ongoing research related to cellular function of the aging brain.

U. S. GOVERNMENT PUBLICATIONS

Birren, James E., et al (Editors). Human Aging: A Biological and Behavioral Study. U. S. Department of Health, Education and Welfare. Publication No. (HSM) 71-9051. Superintendent of Documents. U. S. Government Printing Office. Washington, D. C. 1971.

Gibson, Don C. (Editor). Development of the Rodent as a Model System of Aging. National Institute of Child Health and Human Development. U. S. Department of Health, Education and Welfare. DHEW Publication No. (NIH) 72-121. Superintendent of Documents. U. S. Government Printing Office. Washington, D. C. 1972.

Granick, Samuel, and Patterson, Robert D. (Editors). Human Aging II: An Eleven-Year Followup Biomedical and Behavioral Study. National Institute of Mental Health. Rockville, Maryland. 1971.

Ryan, Kenneth J., and Gibson, Don C. (Editors). Menopause and Aging. National Institute of Child Health and Human Development. U. S. Department of Health, Education and Welfare. DHEW Publication No. (NIH) 73-319. Superintendent of Documents. U. S. Government Printing Office. Washington, D. C. 1973.

AGING, PSYCHOLOGICAL

Ames, Louise Bates, et al. Rorschach Responses in Old Age. Brunner/ Mazel, Inc. New York, New York. 1975.

Report of the results of an extensive Rorschach study of subjects between the ages of 70 years and 100 years.

Barrett, James H. Gerontological Psychology. Charles C. Thomas. Springfield, Illinois. 1972.

Data from an empirical study of 159 older persons, ages 65-100 years, are used to refute stereotypes about the aged and their functional capabilities.

Bell, Benjamin, et al (Editors). Symposium on Personality, Age, and the Social Indices. 81st Annual Convention of the American Psychological Association, 1973. American Psychological Association. Washington, D. C. 1973.

Title self explanatory.

Bengtson, Vern L. The Social Psychology of Aging. The Bobbs-Merrill Company, Inc. Indianapolis, Indiana. 1973.

A study contrasting three generations of a single family, which demonstrates that aging is a function of both time and social process. The nature of adjustments in later years is explored.

Birren, James E. (Editor). Handbook of Aging and the Individual: Psychological and Biological Aspects. The University of Chicago Press. Chicago, Illinois. 1971.

Research findings on biological and psychological bases for changes which occur in the aging individual including behavioral ramifications of change and individual capacities.

________________________. Relations of Stress and Age. The Ethel Percy Andrus Gerontology Center. University of Southern California. Los Angeles, California. 1975.

A bibliography.

Birren, James E. (Editor). The Psychology of Aging. Prentice-Hall, Inc. Englewood Cliffs, New Jersey. 1964.

Based upon research results then available, this book details facts about human aging and the processes of transformation affecting humans during the latter half of life.

________________, and Schaie, K. Warner (Editors). Handbook of the Psychology of Aging. Van Nostrand Reinhold Company. New York, New York. 1977.

Vol. 2 in the Handbooks of Aging Series covers major aspects of the psychology of aging. Background information on research in both psychology of aging and biological aspects of behavior is included.

Bischof, Ledford J. Adult Psychology. Second Edition. Harper and Row Publishers, Inc. New York, New York. 1976.

This new edition includes recent research studies about the period of life from early adulthood to old age.

Botwinick, Jack. Aging and Behavior: A Comprehensive Integration of Research Findings. Springer Publishing Company, Inc. New York, New York. 1973.

Presentation of the psychological processes and changes associated with aging; concludes with a discussion on methodological, operational, and conceptual issues in research.

________________. Cognitive Processes in Maturity and Old Age. Springer Publishing Company. New York, New York. 1967.

A discussion of problems in cognitive functioning with emphasis upon later life functions.

________________ and Storanett, Martha. Memory, Related Functions and Age. Charles C. Thomas. Springfield, Illinois. 1974.

A description of different types of memory and their behavioral correlates.

Boyer, Ruth Gasink. Tomorrow Is Living. The John E. Barton Company. Tallahassee, Florida. 1968.

A subjective review of factors related to successful aging.

Britton, Joseph H. and Britton, Jean O. Personality Changes in Aging: A Longitudinal Study of Community Residents. Springer Publishing Company, Inc. New York, New York. 1972.

A nine-year inquiry into how advancing years affect the average citizen's ability to cope with life stress. The study is relevant for community action programs on behalf of the old, and to behavioral scientists engaged in theoretical and methodological research in gerontology and in social and developmental psychology.

Bromley, D. B. The Psychology of Human Ageing. Second Edition. Penquin Books, Inc. Baltimore, Maryland. 1974.

Topics include: biological and social aspects of aging, personality and psychopathology in adult life, mental disease in old age and adult intelligence.

Burr, Helen Turner (Editor). Psychological Functioning of Older People. Third Edition. Charles C. Thomas. Springfield, Illinois. 1971.

A monograph designed to inform gerontology practioners about needs of the aged and how to meet them.

Butler, Robert N. and Lewis, Myrna I. Aging and Mental Health: Positive Psychosocial Approaches. The C. V. Mosby Company St. Louis, Missouri. 1973.

An extensive coverage of the nature and problems of old age; offers constructive approaches to psychosocial solutions.

Charles, Don C. and Looft, W. R. Readings in Psychological Development Throughout Life. Holt, Rinehart and Winston, Inc. New York, New York. 1973.

Book of readings in the areas of developmental psychology, physiological bases of behavior, social behavior and adjustment.

Datan, Nancy and Ginsberg, Leon H. (Editors). Life-Span Developmental Psychology: Normative Life Crises. Academic Press. New York, New York. 1975.

A compilation of studies on normative life crises ranging from youth through old age, with substantial attention given to later years. Includes contributions from researchers and practitioners from a variety of disciplines.

Erp, Sue H. Aging: Psychological Changes. Oregon Center for Gerontology. Continuing Education Publication. University of Oregon. Corvallis, Oregon. 1972.

Programmed text which provides a practical approach to the psychological dimensions of aging; suitable as a supplementary text.

Eisdorfer, Carl, and Lawton, M. P. (Editors). The Psychology of Adult Development and Aging. American Psychological Association. Washington, D. C. 1973.

A summary report on gerontological research covering a wide range of topics, e.g., education, housing, transportation, and animal research.

Geist, Harold. The Psychological Aspects of the Aging Process, With Sociological Implications. Warren H. Green, Inc. St. Louis, Missouri. 1968.

An elementary textbook covering the aging process with psychological and sociological emphasis.

Gentry, W. Doyle. Geropsychology: A Model of Training and Clinical Service. Ballinger Publishing Company. Cambridge, Massachusetts. 1976.

A book of essays dealing with the role of psychology in health care services for the elderly. It includes also a curriculum for training geropsychologists and an evaluation of the adequacy of current psychological treatment programs.

Goulet, L. R., and Baltes, P. B. (Editors). Life-Span Developmental Psychology: Research and Theory. Academic Press. New York, New York. 1970.

Collection of papers from a conference sponsored by West Virginia University. The 18 chapters range in content from theory and methodology to presentations of research in perception, learning, retention, language, and cognitive abilities as they relate to the life-span.

Gutmann, David L. The Country of Old Men: Cultural Studies in the Psychology of Later Life. Occasional Papers in Gerontology. Institute of Gerontology. University of Michigan. Ann Arbor, Michigan. 1969.

An examination of questions related to the psychology of aging among those in pre-literate Indian societies.

Harris, Louis, and Associates. The Myth and Reality of Aging in America. National Council on the Aging, Inc. Washington, D. C. 1975.

A 245 page report of an attitudinal study of old age, including both general public and aged persons themselves. Implications for public policy are extensive.

Heron, Alastair, and Chown, Sheila. Age and Function. Little, Brown and Company. Boston, Massachusetts. 1967.

Description of the extensive variations among healthy old people with regard to personality, perception, and performance, and the wide differences within individuals in rate of change for various functions.

Hulicka, Irene M. Empirical Studies in the Psychology and Sociology of Aging. Thomas Y. Crowell Company. New York, New York. 1977.

A compilation of abstracts of 140 papers on the study of aging, with selections based upon the importance assigned to the area of research, the research design, results obtained and potential effects.

Jarvik, Lissy F., et al (Editors). Intellectual Functioning in Adults: Psychological and Biological Influences. Springer Publishing Company. New York, New York. 1973.

Report of studies from the second through the ninth decade of life concerning psychological and biological influences on intellectual functioning; delineates problems in such research, and suggests prospects for developmental research.

Kalish, Richard A. (Editor). The Dependencies of Old People. Institute of Gerontology. The University of Michigan-Wayne State University. Ann Arbor, Michigan. August, 1969.

Exploration of the psychodynamics of the dependencies of old people.

__________________. Late Adulthood: Perspectives on Human Development. Brooks/Cole Publishing Company. Monterey, California. 1975.

Attention is centered upon the psychology of late maturity and old age.

Kaluger, George, and Kaluger, Meriem Fair. *Profiles in Human Development*. The C. V. Mosby Company. St. Louis, Missouri. 1976.

A text that utilizes brief narratives to further understanding of life experiences at different stages in development. Special emphasis is given to adult life, including old age.

Kuhlen, R. G., et al. *Syracuse University Bibliography: Learning and Cognitive Performance in Adults*. Syracuse University Press. Syracuse, New York. 1967.

A reference resource on adult psychological performances.

Levin, Sidney, and Kahana, Ralph J. (Editors). *Psychodynamic Studies on Aging: Creativity, Reminiscing and Dying*. International Universities Press. New York, New York. 1967.

The reports challenge the idea that creativity decreases with age.

Lewis, Edwin C., et al. *The Psychology of Human Development: A Life-Span Approach*. The Dryden Press. Hinsdale, Illinois. 1975.

A text for developmental psychology with emphasis upon cognitive and biological development. Coverage extends into adulthood and old age.

Lidz, Theodore. *The Person*. (Revised) Basic Books, Inc. New York, New York. 1976.

A recognized text on personality development throughout the life cycle, which now includes expanded sections on middle years and old age.

Maas, Henry, and Kuypers, Joseph. *From Thirty to Seventy*. Jossey-Bass, Inc. San Francisco, California. 1974.

Report of a 40-year longitudinal study of adult life styles and personalities, providing reliable information about middle class adult life and documenting continuity rather than change over the years.

Neugarten, Bernice L., et al. _Personality in Middle and Late Life._ Atherton Press. New York, New York. 1964.

Report on eight studies relating various psychological approaches to personality.

Newman, Barbara M., and Newman, Philip R. _Development Through Life: A Psychosocial Approach._ The Dorsey Press. Homewood, Illinois. 1975.

This book concerns normal development throughout life, tracing significant changes at each period of life. Emphasis is given to changes in intellect, emotions and social relationships.

________________________________. _Development Through Life: A Case Study Approach._ The Dorsey Press. Homewood, Illinois. 1975.

This is a companion resource book to _Development Through Life: A Psychosocial Approach._ For each stage of life, selections are given based on autobiographies, letters, diaries, interviews and other sources, including traditional psychological case materials.

Niebanck, Paul L., and Pope, John B. _The Elderly in Older Urban Areas: Problems of Adaptation and the Effects of Relocation._ Institute for Environmental Studies. University of Pennsylvania. Philadelphia, Pennsylvania. 1965.

Description of characteristics of relocated elderly persons and the general impact of such a transition upon them. Discussion of programs and ideas for programs to improve the relocation process are included.

Nydegger, Corinne, et al. _Measurements of Morale._ The Gerontological Society. Washington, D. C. 1977.

This monograph deals with the measurement of factors that affect individual functioning, and practical approaches to better morale through improved functioning.

Pastalan, Leon A., and Carson, Daniel H. (Editors). Spatial Behavior of Older People. Institute of Gerontology. University of Michigan-Wayne State University. University of Michigan Press. Ann Arbor, Michigan. 1970.

A discussion of research involving the observation and study of spatial allocations among the elderly.

Psychosocial Needs of the Aged, The. Ethel Percy Andrus Gerontology Center. University of Southern California. Los Angeles, California. 1973.

This monograph is designed for those who deliver services to the elderly, especially nursing care and social service. It is divided into three sections, namely, needs, care and training.

Savage, R. D., et al (Editors). Intellectual Functioning in the Aged. Methuen Press. London, England. 1973, and Harper and Row Publishers, Inc. New York, New York. 1975.

A manual of modern psychology dealing with the psychological and intellectual functioning of the aged.

Schaie, K. Warner (Editor). Intellectual Functioning and Aging. The Ethel Percy Andrus Gerontology Center. University of Southern California. Los Angeles, California. 1975.

A bibliography.

________________________. Theory and Methods of Research in Aging. West Virginia University. Morgantown, West Virginia. 1968.

Composite of conference papers dealing primarily with psychological aspects of aging.

Schwartz, Arthur N. (Editor). Psychological Adjustment to Aging. The Ethel Percy Andrus Gerontology Center. University of Southern California. Los Angeles, California. 1975.

A bibliography.

Seabrook, Jeremy. Loneliness. Universe Books. New York, New York. 1975.

Report on a series of interviews which contribute insight on loneliness. A number of these interviews were conducted among middle-aged and older people.

Selye, Hans. The Stress of Life. Revised Edition. McGraw-Hill Book Company. New York, New York. 1976.

This revised and expanded edition of the 1956 book is written by a major authority on the stress theory. Attention is given to stress effects throughout life.

Silverman, Phyllis R., et al (Editors). Helping Each Other in Widowhood. Health Sciences Publishing Corporation. New York, New York. 1974.

A collection of workshop reports dealing with the emotional and mental health aspects of widowhood. Emphasis is upon the widow-to-widow program as a preventive measure to lessen emotional trauma.

Simon, Alexander, and Epstein, Leon J. (Editors). Aging in Modern Society. (Psychiatric Research Report No. 23). American Psychiatric Association. Washington, D. C. 1968.

Conference papers on the general topic of aging and societal impact.

Simon, Anne W. The New Years: A New Middle Age. Alfred A. Knopf. New York, New York. 1968.

This book claims that intelligence is not impaired with age and that aging men and women are capable of and eager to perform in creative work.

Talland, G. A. (Editor). Human Behavior and Aging. Academic Press. New York, New York. 1968.

An examination of specific tasks performed by older persons, and the presentation of a derived theory correlating aging and behavior.

Thomas, H., et al (Editors). Patterns of Aging: Findings from the Bonn Longitudinal Study of Aging. S. Karger. Basel, Switzerland. 1976.

The first report of this study begun in 1965 in Bonn University includes subjects in West Germany born between 1890 and 1895 and 1900-1905. The topics covered include: cognitive functioning, psychomotor performance, personality, ecology and adjustment, social roles, leisure, and successful aging.

Vedder, Clyde B., and Lefkowitz, Annette S. (Editors). Problems of the Aged. Charles C. Thomas. Springfield, Illinois. 1965.

Discussions of the frustrations and anxieties among the aged and how they might be alleviated.

Welford, A. T., and Birren, James E. (Editors). Decision Making and Age. Interdisciplinary Topics in Gerontology, Vol. 4. NATO Advanced Study Institute. University of Thessaloniki, August 14-19, 1967. S. Karger. New York, New York. 1969.

A collection of cross-cultural studies on decision making among the aged.

Wolk, Robert L., and Wolk, Rochelle B. The Gerontological Apperception Test. Behavioral Publications, Inc. New York, New York. (N.D.)

A projective test for use in personality study of old people. This is modification of the TAT which uses themes and situations more common to old people.

Atchley, Robert C. The Social Forces in Later Life: An Introduction to Social Gerontology. Second Edition. Wadsworth Publishing Company, Inc. Belmont, California. 1977.

A good survey text in the area of aging.

Baum, D. J. The Final Plateau. Burns and McEachern. Toronto, Ontario, Canada. (N.D.)

This book gives an overview of aging in Canada; deals with societal problems and needs.

Beard, Belle Boone. Social Competence of Centenarians. University of Georgia Printing Department. Athens, Georgia. 1967.

Report on an empirical study of centenarians in the United States.

Bell, Bill D. (Editor). Contemporary Social Gerontology. Charles C. Thomas. Springfield, Illinois. 1976.

Significant developments in the field of aging.

Bengtson, V. L., and Laufer, R. S. (Editors). "Youth, Generations and Social Change," Journal of Social Sciences, Vol. 30, Part I. The Society for the Psychological Study of Social Issues. American Psychological Association. Ann Arbor, Michigan. 1974.

A compilation of analyses of the age-old problem of generations and social change. Emphasis is upon social movements and contrasting youth and the aged.

Binstock, Robert H. (Editor). Handbook of Aging and the Social Sciences. Van Nostrand Reinhold Company. New York, New York. 1977.

The first volume in the Handbooks of Aging Series is a comprehensive examination of biological, psychological and social ramifications of aging.

Brearley, C. Paul. Social Work, Ageing and Society. Routledge and Kegan Paul. Boston, Massachusetts. 1975.

The author emphasizes the needs of old people and their worth in society, and reviews social attitudes. Could be useful to students in social work or other caring professions.

Buckley, Mary. The Aged Are People Too: About William Posner and Social Work With the Old. Introduction by Arthur S. Faber. National University Publications. Kinnikat Press. Port Washington, New York. 1972.

An account of the achievements of William Posner and of his contributions to the field of social work through his work with aged persons. Includes a bibliography of Posner's publications.

Clark, Margaret and Anderson, Barbara G. Culture and Aging. Charles C. Thomas. Springfield, Illinois. 1967.

The authors give a socio-cultural perspective to problems of the aged in the United States. Reports research data obtained from 435 older persons, including those living normal, adjusted lives in the community and others with a history of psychiatric illness.

Cottrell, Fred. Aging and the Aged. William C. Brown Company. Dubuque, Iowa. 1974.

A consideration of aging within a sociological framework. Topics included are: processes of aging, health, income, employment, retirement, social and political participation, family, religion, government and non-government organizations.

Cumming, E. and Henry, W. Growing Old: The Process of Disengagement. Basic Books. New York, New York. 1961.

An early pioneer publication which treats aging as a psycho-social phenomenon. Based upon observations in a midwestern town, the conclusions reached described the older persons as "disengaging" from previous life activities.

Eisele, Frederick R. "Political Consequences of Aging." The Annals of the American Academy of Political and Social Science. Vol. 415. September, 1974.

A special volume of the Annals devoted to issues in public policy, political behavior, and the political future related to the aged.

Gubrium, Jaber F. The Myth of the Golden Years: A Socio-Environmental Theory of Aging. Charles C. Thomas. Springfield, Illinois. 1972.

Explorations of current theories of aging; emphasizing the socioenvironmental approach as a viable theory.

________________. Time, Roles, and Self in Old Age. Behavioral Publications, Inc. New York, New York. 1975.

A resource book in gerontology which deals with such topics as politics of age, the world of the single elderly, the meaning of the generation gap, the effect upon self of consistency in roles, and how people respond to time-disordered relationships. Retirement is discussed as it affects attitudes and behavior.

Hazell, Kenneth. Social and Medical Problems of the Elderly. Third Edition. Charles C. Thomas. Springfield, Illinois. 1973.

Emphasis is given to hospital care of aged patients, although considerable attention is given to social problems of the aged in England. This book has special value to practitioners in the health care field.

Hochschild, Arlie Russell. The Unexpected Community. Prentice-Hall. Englewood Cliffs, New Jersey. 1973.

Examination of the life style of old people living in a small apartment building in the San Francisco Bay area.

Holtzman, Abraham. The Townsend Movement; A Political Study. Bookman Associates. New York, New York. 1963.

An analysis of the movement initiated by Dr. Francis Townsend, which was designed to help people who needed assistance prior to the passage of the Social Security Act. Valuable reference to historical perspective.

Jacobs, Jerry. Older Persons and Retirement Communities. Charles C. Thomas. Springfield, Illinois. 1975.

These case studies in social gerontology have sought to investigate the everyday life of older retired persons and to accumulate descriptive data necessary for ethnographic study. Techniques employed were informal interview and direct observation.

Kart, Cary S. and Manard, Barbara. Aging in America: Readings in Social Gerontology. Alfred Publishing Company, Inc. Port Washington, New York. 1976.

A book of readings in social gerontology divided into seven major sections:

I. Theoretical Approaches to Social Aging
II. Methodological Issues in Social Gerontology
III. Biological and Psychological Aspects of Aging
IV. Work, Retirement and Leisure
V. Living Environments
VI. Institutionalization
VII. Death and Dying

Kleyman, Paul. Senior Power: Growing Old Rebelliously. Glide Publications. San Francisco, California. 1974.

Suggested political action for the aged drawn from the experiences of the California Legislative Council for Older Americans.

Loether, Herman J. Problems of Aging: Sociological and Social Psychological Perspectives. Second Edition. Dickenson Publishing Company, Inc. Encino, California. 1975.

Brief monograph covering such areas as understanding the aging process, interpersonal relations, health, housing, employment and exploitation of the aged.

Niebanck, Paul L. and Yessian, Mark R. Relocation in Urban Planning: From Obstacle to Opportunity. University of Pennsylvania Press. Philadelphia, Pennsylvania. 1968.

Discussion of increasing problems associated with displacement of the elderly in urban renewal areas.

Puner, Morton. To the Good Long Life. Universe Books. New York, New York. 1974.

A book on the aging process and what it means to be elderly in today's society; written for lay audience.

Pollak, Otto and Heathers, Glen. Social Adjustment in Old Age: A Research Planning Report. Greenwood Press. Westport, Connecticut. 1975.

A reprint of the 1948 edition, which was published by the Social Science Research Council. Covers the status and role of the aged in the United States with attention directed toward social adjustment.

Rose, Arnold, M. and Peterson, Warren O. (Editors). Older People and Their Social World: The Subculture of the Aging. F. A. Davis. Philadelphia, Pennsylvania. 1965.

An anthology in social gerontology reflecting use of a variety of social research techniques in studies reported.

Rosenberg, G. S. The Worker Grows Old. Jossey-Bass, Inc., Publishers. San Francisco, California. 1970.

This book explores the relationship between poverty and old age and between poverty and isolation of the aged and compares the more affluent aged to the poor. There is also some discussion of the beliefs and attitudes of the aged on isolation, old age, and social class.

Rosow, Irving. Social Integration of the Aged. The Free Press. New York, New York. 1967.

An analysis of the obstacles and opportunities which determine the quality and quantity of social participation of the aged.

____________. Socialization to Old Age. University of California Press. Berkeley, California. 1975.

An analysis of socialization to old age with suggested ways to facilitate the development of appropriate old age norms and roles.

Rudd, T. N. Human Relations in Old Age. Faber. London, England. 1967.

A handbook for persons in service occupations whose work brings them in contact with the aged.

Shanas, Ethel, et al. <u>Old People in Three Industrial Societies</u>. Atherton Press. New York, New York. 1968.

Report on a cross-national survey of living conditions and behavior of elderly people in Denmark, Britain, and the United States.

Silverman, Phyllis R., et al. (Editors). <u>Helping Each Other in Widowhood</u>. Health Sciences Publishing Corp. New York, New York. 1974.

Proceedings from two workshops sponsored by the Widow-to-Widow Program at Harvard Medical School. The first workshop provided an opportunity for widows and widowers to share experiences. The second was designed to inform professional workers of the needs of the widowed.

Simpson, Ida Harper and McKinney, John C. (Editors). <u>Social Aspects of Aging</u>. Duke University Press. Durham, N.C. 1966.

Report of a series of pilot studies covering economic and related determinants affecting older worker occupational role; work and retirement; family and retirement; community; self-orientation.

Tibbitts, Clark (Editor). <u>Handbook of Social Gerontology: Societal Aspects of Aging</u>. The University of Chicago Press. Chicago, Illinois. 1960.

One of the earlier publications in the field, this handbook, part two of a series, provides material useful in training scientists and professional personnel in social gerontology. Compiled by the integrated efforts of 23 scholars, it provides comprehensive reading in this field.

______________ and Donahue, Wilma (Editors). <u>Social and Psychological Aspects of Aging</u>. Columbia University Press. New York, New York. 1968.

Subject content covers a broad spectrum of social aspects and psychological studies of aged individuals, as well as group behavior and social action around the world. The several components are brought together in critical review by the editors.

Tunstall, Jeremy. Old and Alone; A Sociological Study of Old People. Routledge and Kegan-Paul, Ltd. London, England. 1966.

Examination of the meanings of aloneness among the aged; defines four categories of aloneness.

Twente, Esther E. Never Too Old. Jossey-Bass, Inc. San Francisco, California. 1970.

The focus is upon aged persons in small communities and their group identity.

Vischer, A. L. On Growing Old. Houghton Mifflin, Co. Boston, Massachusetts. 1967.

A discussion of old people in relation to their past life and experiences and to their present social environment.

Williams, Richard H. and Wirths, Claudine G. Lives Through the Years: Styles of Life and Successful Aging. Atherton Press. New York, New York. 1965.

Report based upon intensive interviews with older persons. The authors relate life styles to successful aging. The emphasis is upon correlation of the degree of success in aging adaptations in the continuation of established life style.

Youmans, E. G. (Editor). Older Rural Americans: A Sociological Perspective. University of Kentucky Press. Lexington, Kentucky. 1967.

A study of older rural residents in the context of work, family and community. Analyzes geographical distribution and economic, health and housing status. Special attention is given to older populations who are American Indian, Negro and those in the Southwestern United States.

U. S. GOVERNMENT PUBLICATIONS

Coelho, George V., and Rubinstein, Eli A. (Editors). Social Change and Human Behavior: Mental Health Challenges of the Seventies. U. S. Department of Health, Education and Welfare. Public Health Services. National Institute of Mental Health. Rockville, Maryland. 1972.

Sherman, Edith M., and Britton, Margaret R. Patterns for Progress in Aging: Work Study in Social Gerontology, Demonstration Project at University of Denver. Administration on Aging. U. S. Department of Health, Education and Welfare. DHEW Publication No. (SRS) 73-20190. Superintendent of Documents. U. S. Government Printing Office. Washington, D. C. 1973.

Social Services, Aging, Retirement, and Social Welfare. Public Documents Department. Superintendent of Documents. U. S. Government Printing Office. Washington, D. C. 1973.

CHURCH AND RELIGION

Bentley, Virgil. *The Beauty of Age: Biblical Themes on Aging for Young and Old.* Gospel Teachers Publications, Inc. Dallas, Texas. 1975.

A compilation of sermons on aging designed to encourage clergymen to deal with the subject. Includes a scriptural index and a brief annotated bibliography.

Bier, William C. *Aging: Its Challenge to the Individual and Society.* Fordham University Press. New York, New York. 1974.

Published proceedings of the eight biennial institutes in Pastoral Psychology at Fordham University. Special attention is given to the place of religion in gerontology, but the materials are basically an overview of the field of aging.

Brown, J. Paul. *Counseling with Senior Citizens.* Prentice-Hall, Inc. Englewood Cliffs, New Jersey. 1964.

Based on personal experiences of the author, this work is offered as an aid to the clergyman in working with older people.

Clingan, Donald F. *Aging Persons in the Community of Faith.* The Author. P. O. Box 1986. Indianapolis, Indiana. 46206. 1975.

An interfaith guidebook for ministry with aged persons. It includes the needs of the aged and the roles of congregations and communities in meeting these needs.

Ellison, Jerome. *The Last Third of Life Club.* United Church Press. Philadelphia, Pennsylvania. 1973.

Explanation of the purposes and objectives of the Last Third of Life Club, an organization concerned with the religious aspects of retirement years.

Grey Sisters. *Strategy for Tomorrow's Living.* (Extracts from Program, Dynamics of Retirement, July 4-9, 1971.) Grey Sisters Motherhouse. Pembroke, Ontario, Canada. 1971.

Report of a seminar on retirement, health, nutrition and spiritual accomodation to the aging process.

Guide to Aging Programs. Synagogue Council of America. Washington, D. C. 1975.

A ninety-six page guide describing why synagogues should organize to meet the needs of the elderly Jewish population, and offering procedures for doing so.

Hiltner, Seward (Editor). Toward a Theology of Aging. Human Sciences Press. New York, New York. 1975.

A volume of essays based upon lectures given in May, 1974, at the Kansas City Conference on Aging, sponsored by the National Retired Teachers Association and the American Association of Retired Persons. The essays cover psychological, socio-historical and theological meanings of aging in human life.

Kutscher, Austin H., and Kutscher, Lillian G. (Editors). Religion and Bereavement: Counsel for the Physician; Advice for the Bereaved; Thoughts for the Clergyman. Health Sciences Publishing Corporation. New York, New York. 1972.

Based upon the Judao-Christian traditions, the book offers counsel for self understanding as well as understanding of others.

Mow, Anna B. So Who's Afraid of Birthdays. J. B. Lippincott Company. Philadelphia, Pennsylvania. 1969.

Reflections on growing old graciously with emphasis upon opportunities for spiritual growth in the retirement years.

Robb, Thomas Bradley. The Bonus Years: Foundations for Ministry with Older Persons. The Judson Press. Valley Forge, Pennsylvania. 1968.

Very simply written, the first few chapters describe characteristics and problems of the aged, and later chapters consider the role of the church in meeting needs among the elderly. Program initiation and implementation is considered.

Ruoss, Meryl. Citizen Power and Social Change: The Challenge to Churches. Seabury Press. New York, New York. 1968.

A discussion of the role of the church in working with citizen organizations to achieve social change.

That Thy Days May Be Long in the Good Land: A Guide For Aging Programs For Synagogues. Synagogue Council of America. New York, New York. 1975.

A guidebook for planning, developing and operating programs and services for the aged.

Tournier, Paul. The Seasons of Life. John Knox Press. Richmond, Virginia. 1972.

The life cycle of man is compared to the seasons of nature.

Vandenburgh, Mildred. Fill Your Days With Life. Royal Books. Glendale, California. 1975.

A book devoted to the content of life with a special emphasis on the religious life of the aged.

U.S. GOVERNMENT PUBLICATIONS

Brighter Vistas: Church Programs for Older Adults. DHEW Pub. No. (OHD) 74-20188. Administration on Aging. Department of Health, Eduation and Welfare. Washington, D.C. 1965.

Spiritual Well-Being. 1971 White House Conference on Aging. Superintendent of Documents. U.S. Government Printing Office. Washington, D.C. 1972.

Stough, Ada Barnett. Brighter Vistas: The Story of Four Church Programs for Older Adults. AoA No. 18. Superintendent of Documents. U.S. Government Printing Office. Washington, D.C. 1965.

What Churches Can Do: Interfaith Opportunity Center. U.S. Department of Health, Education and Welfare. Social and Rehabilitation Service. Administration on Aging. U.S. Government Printing Office. Washington, D.C. September, 1968.

What Churches Can Do: Satellite Housing Projects. U.S. Department of Health, Education and Welfare. Social and Rehabilitation Services. Administration on Aging. AoA Publication No. 900. Superintendent of Documents. U.S. Government Printing Office. Washington, D.C. April, 1968.

COMMUNITY AND SOCIAL SERVICES

Agency Self-Evaluation Guides for Serving Older People. American Public Welfare Association. Public Welfare Project on Aging. Chicago, Illinois. 1965.

Title self explanatory. This small publication is old, but offers helpful information.

Barney, Jane Lockwood. *The Well-Being Report: A Look at Supportive Services for the Elderly*. Institute of Gerontology. University of Michigan-Wayne State University. Ann Arbor, Michigan. 1975.

A report on the first 10 years of the Well-Being Service for Aging in Detroit, Michigan, designed to assist elderly persons to continue their independence. Includes the history of the service, characteristics of clients, needs and services.

Bell, Duran, et al. *Delivering Services to Elderly Members of Minority Groups: A Critical Review of the Literature*. Publications Department. The Rand Corporation. Santa Monica, California. 1976.

A broad spectrum of services is included and the principal problems are identified, according to conclusions by the authors. Corrective recommendations are made. Sponsor of the study was the Administration on Aging, Office of Human Development, U. S. Department of Health, Education and Welfare.

Bloom, Jane E. *Revenue Sharing and the Elderly: How to Play and Win*. The National Council on the Aging, Inc. Washington, D. C. 1973.

A guidebook for agencies serving the elderly on how to obtain monies under the Title I Revenue Sharing Act.

———————— and Cohen, Robert H. *Social Services for the Elderly: Funding Projects in Model Cities Through Titles I and XVI of the Social Security Act*. The National Council on the Aging and National Leagues of Cities. U. S. Conference of Mayors. Washington, D. C. 1972.

Guidelines for cities and communities interested in developing and funding social service programs for the aged.

Brearley, C. Paul. Social Work, Aging and Society. Routledge and Kegan Paul. Boston, Massachusetts. 1975.

The author emphasizes the needs of the elderly, together with the role of old persons in society and current attitudes toward them. Affirms that work with the aged is both interesting and worthwhile.

Brody, Elaine M. Long-Term Care of Older People: A Practical Guide. Human Sciences Press. New York, New York. 1977.

This book concerns aged persons in the community and in various types of institutions. The four sections of the volume are: an historical perspective and current status in long-term care; social aspects of care; institutions; and family.

Brown, Ruth E. Community Action Programs: An Annotated Bibliography. Council of Planning Librarians. Monticello, Illinois. 1972.

A compilation of resources about initiation and implementation of community action agencies, the role and function of boards of directors, and the effect of programs on the community.

Brudney, Juliet F. The Janus Project: Advocacy and Service for the Elderly Relocatee. Institute for Environmental Studies. University of Pennsylvania. Philadelphia, Pennsylvania. 1969.

Suggestions given of the kinds of help that can be provided to assist relocated aged persons.

Buckley, Many. The Aged are People, Too. Kennikat Press. Port Washington, New York. 1972.

A book about William Posner and his social work with the aged. Has value both for agency structure and service practices and for professional workers with the aged.

Carter, Beryl, and Siegel, Sheldon. An Annotated Selective Bibliography for Social Work with the Aging. Council on Social Work Education. New York, New York. 1968.

A bibliography of periodical articles covering the period 1959-1967 and compiled especially for social workers and students. Covers references pertaining to methods and techniques, programs and services.

Chandler, Suzannah. *A Comprehensive Program for the Elderly in Rural Areas*. Revised. National Council on the Aging. Washington, D. C. 1972.

Title self explanatory.

_______________. *Home Maintenance and Repair Program for the Older Poor*. A Model Community Action Program. National Council on the Aging. New York, New York. 1968.

Report on maintenance repair service program for the elderly with the repairs being made by persons in need of employment.

Collins, Alice H., and Pancoast, Diane L. *Natural Helping Networks: A Strategy for Prevention*. National Association of Social Workers. Washington, D. C. 1976.

Utilization of resources is dealt with, emphasizing needed and available support systems.

Community Care Programs for the Elderly. Committee on Aging. Community Service Society of New York. 105 East 22nd Street. New York, New York. 1976.

This publication consists of three sections. One section gives background information on aging and on mental health; the second is a report on the symposium on "New Ideas for Alternatives to Institutional Care for the Elderly;" and the third section is a description of 37 programs in New York City which emphasize services to frail elderly.

Communication Skills for the Gerontological Practitioner. Gerontology Center. Institute for the Study of Human Development. Pennsylvania State University. University Park, Pennsylvania. 1976.

Emphasis in this manual is placed on the importance of person-to-person communication in the delivery of human services. Examples and exercises are drawn from the field of gerontology.

Continuing Choices: A Comprehensive Handbook of Programs for Work With Older Adults. National Council of Jewish Women. New York, New York. 1975.

A handbook which not only suggests ways to provide services to the elderly, but also how to utilize the energy and experience of older Americans in doing so.

Davenhall, William F. _Rural Home Repair: A Local, State, and Federal Demonstration_. Spindletop Research, Inc. Lexington, Kentucky. 1973.

An evaluation report on the Eastern Kentucky Rural Home Improvement demonstration project. Home repairs were made for public assistance clients using Office of Economic Opportunity labor. A majority of the homes were those of aged, blind, or disabled clients.

Day Care for the Elderly and _Working With the Elderly_. 2 Volume Set. Institute of Gerontology. University of Michigan. Ann Arbor, Michigan. 1975.

Annotated bibliography on the subjects specified.

Edwards, M. I. _Selected References on Meals-On-Wheels Service_. Institute of Gerontology. Iowa University. Iowa City, Iowa. 1966.

An annotated bibliography.

Evaluation of the Foster Grandparent Program, An. Greenleigh Associates. New York, New York. 1966.

An evaluation of the Foster Grandparent Program from the experience of 10 local or state-wide projects.

Fowler, Talmadge. _Alternatives to the Single Site Center_. The National Council on the Aging. Washington, D. C. 1974.

An excellent resource for agency heads seeking information about the development or expansion of service delivery networks for the elderly in a community; discusses interagency and agency linkages.

Hardy, Richard E., and Cull, John G. _Organization and Administration of Service Programs for the Older American_. Charles C. Thomas. Springfield, Illinois. 1975.

Description of a sample of service programs available to aged Americans; intended audience includes both professionals and older Americans themselves.

Home Delivered Meals. National Council on the Aging. Washington, D. C. (N.D.)

A bibliography.

Home Maintenance and Repair Program for the Older Poor. National Council on Aging. Washington, D. C. 1972.

A simple publication designed to give guidelines for a home support service for the elderly.

Human Services and Social Work Responsibility. Professional Sumposium on Human Services and Professional Responsibility. National Association of Social Workers. New York, New York. 1969.

Definition of the roles of professionals and non-professionals, social agencies, senior centers and community organizations in the effective delivery of needed human services.

Jeffers, Frances C. (Editor). Guidelines for an Information and Counseling Service for Older Persons. Center for the Study of Aging and Human Development, Duke University. Durham, North Carolina. 1970.

Subjects covered include organization and operation of a multi-disciplinary service agency designed to meet needs of older persons.

Kell, Jeffrey. Joint Project for Rural Home Repair: A Cooperative Demonstration Project Stimulated Through Section 1115 of the Social Security Act. Spindletop Research. Lexington, Kentucky. 1970.

Analysis and evaluation of a demonstration project to repair rural homes.

Lawton, M. Powell, et al (Editors). Community Planning for an Aging Society. Dowden, Hutchinson & Ross, Inc. Stroudsburg, Pennsylvania. 1976.

An analysis of assets, liabilities and needs of older persons, and an exploration of important considerations pertinent in planning facilities and services.

Lawton, M. Powell, and Byerts, Thomas (Editors). <u>Community Planning for the Elderly</u>. The Gerontological Society. Washington, D. C. 1973.

A compilation of findings from research and experience associated with urban physical planning and program development for the elderly.

__________________. <u>Social and Medical Services in Housing for the Aged</u>. Philadelphia Geriatric Center. Philadelphia, Pennsylvania. 1968.

A study of 1800 tenants or applicants for housing for the elderly. Some were interviewed before moving and some afterwards.

Long, Nicholas. <u>Information and Referral Centers: A Functional Analysis</u>. Institute for Interdisciplinary Studies. American Rehabilitation Foundation. Minneapolis, Minnesota. 1971.

Examination of the functions of an information and referral service, and the potential role for such centers in services delivery.

<u>Long-Term Care Handbook: A Description of the Alternative Modes of Health and Health-Related Care for the Elderly and Disabled in Nebraska</u>. Bureau of Comprehensive Health Planning. Nebraska Department of Health. Lincoln, Nebraska. 1975.

A handbook for use by communities in recognizing deficiencies in health care facilities and programs, designed to reduce expense of health care while improving the quality. A section is devoted to each type of long-term care.

Match, Sondra K. (Editor). <u>Community Organization, Planning and Resources and the Older Poor</u>. Senior Opportunities and Services. Technical Assistance Monograph No. 1. National Council on the Aging. Washington, D. C. 1970.

A collection of papers which suggest strategies for organizing older citizens who have limited financial resources to contribute to community planning and action in their own behalf.

__________________. <u>Establishing Telephone Reassurance Service</u>. Senior Opportunities and Services. Technical Assistance Monograph No. 14. National Council on the Aging. Office of Economic Opportunity. Washington, D. C. July, 1972.

Title self explanatory.

Meals on Wheels Manual. Lutheran Service Society of Western Pennsylvania. Pittsburgh, Pennsylvania. 1973.

A practical guide for organizing and operating a Meals-on-Wheels program.

Media and the Elderly, The. National Council on the Aging. Washington, D. C. 1973.

Report of the results of a NCOA study of ways in which TV, radio, and related media can better meet the needs of middle aged and older persons.

More Than Shelter: A Guide to the Development of Community Services for the Aging in Housing Projects in New York State. New York State Interdepartmental Health and Hospital Council. Albany, New York. 1965.

A monograph on the specific subject stated, but with applicability for older persons living elsewhere.

Planning with the Aging: A Process Approach. Syracuse University School of Social Work. Senior Opportunities and Services. Technical Assistance Monograph, No. 6. National Council on the Aging. Washington, D. C. 1971.

Essentials discussed for planning community action programs are: 1) understanding the elderly, and 2) construction of an effective process for service delivery.

Podula, Helen. _Developing Day Care for Older People_. Technical Assistance Monograph: Senior Opportunities and Services, No. 11. National Council on the Aging. Washington, D. C. 1972.

This monograph gives historical perspectives for day care programs. Contents cover definitions, programs, transportation, operation of facilities, safety standards, records, finance, staff, among other topics.

Putter, H., and Malzberg, A. _Helping to Serve the Aging in Their Own Homes: The Effectiveness of Information and Referral Services for Meeting Home Health and Housing Needs of Aging Persons_. Community Council of Greater New York. New York, New York. 1969.

Title self explanatory.

Rachlis, David. Mini-Cost Programs and Services for the Aging Poor. National Council on the Aging. New York, New York. 1969.

A report on the experiences of community agencies and organizations that have developed low cost programs for the aged poor.

Report of the Home Health and Housing Program, Citizens Committee on Aging: January, 1967, Through December, 1969. Community Council of Greater New York. New York, New York. 1970.

Summary of findings and recommendations based upon a three year project to expand home health and housing for the aging.

Report on Services to the Aged. Jewish Federation of Metropolitan Chicago. Chicago, Illinois. 1966.

Discussion of institutional and non-institutional services to Jewish aged with a brief supplement on governmental programs.

Resources for the Aging: An Action Handbook. Second Edition. National Council on the Aging. New York, New York. 1969.

Resource book for alleviating problems of aged poor through use of public and private funds.

Roberts, Nesta. Our Future Selves: Care of the Elderly. Allen and Unwin, Limited. London, England. 1970.

An analysis of the development of services for the elderly with particular attention to the early work of the National Old People's Welfare Council of Great Britain in 1940.

Schulberg, Herbert C., et al (Editors). Developments in Human Services. Vol. 1. Behavioral Publications. New York, New York. 1973.

A textbook, compiled from four monographs, covering service delivery programs and research.

Serving the Urban Elderly: Strategies for Mayors. Prepared by National Conference of Mayors Task Force on Aging. U. S. Conference of Mayors. 1620 Eye Street, N. W. Washington, D. C. 20006.

This volume gives an overview of the status of urban aged and considers the role of cities and their mayors in providing services.

Sinick, Daniel. Counseling Older Persons: Careers, Retirement, Dying. Human Sciences Press. New York, New York. 1977.

As the title indicates, this book offers advice to those counseling the aged in the areas of careers, retirement, and terminal illness.

Sterne, R. S., et al. The Urban Elderly Poor. Lexington Books. Lexington, Massachusetts. 1974.

Emphasis is upon Federally funded Model City Programs in a critical evaluation of the worth of programs designed to help the aged. Analysis of failures is given.

Wasser, Edna. Casebook on Work With the Aging. Family Service Association of America. New York, New York. 1966.

A compilation of ten case studies from the Family Service Association of America's project on aging.

Weisman, Celia B. The Future is Now. National Jewish Welfare Board. New York, New York. 1976.

A manual for programs for elderly persons in Jewish Community Service agencies. The first part concerns a knowledge base for programming, and the second part with program development and types of programs.

Well-Being Report, The. Institute of Gerontology. University of Michigan. Ann Arbor, Michigan. 1975.

Report on a Detroit agency program of providing supportive services to aged persons. Directed to those interested in alternatives to nursing home care.

U. S. GOVERNMENT PUBLICATIONS

Action Act of 1972 and Action Domestic Programs. Labor and Public Welfare Committee, Ninety-second Congress. Second Session. U. S. Senate. Superintendent of Documents. U. S. Government Printing Office. Washington, D. C. 1972.

Buchholtz, Fredric. *Home Delivered Meals for Older Americans.* Administration on Aging. U. S. Department of Health, Education and Welfare. DHEW Publication No. (SRS) 73-20234. Superintendent of Documents. U. S. Government Printing Office. Washington, D. C. 1973.

Comprehensive Care Services in Your Community. U. S. Public Health Service. Publication No. 1353. Superintendent of Documents. U. S. Government Printing Office. Washington, D. C. 1967.

Cushing, Martha, and Long, Nicholas. *Information and Referral Services: Reaching Out.* Administration on Aging. U. S. Department of Health, Education and Welfare. DHEW Publication No. (SRS) 73-20110. Superintendent of Documents. U. S. Government Printing Office. Washington, D. C. 1973.

Day on Wheels. General Services Administration. Public Buildings Service. Washington, D. C. 1975.

Developments and Trends in State Programs and Services for the Elderly. A Survey of Activities at the State Governmental Level in the Field of Aging, 1972 and 1973. A Report to the Special Committee on Aging. United States Senate. Superintendent of Documents. U. S. Government Printing Office. Washington, D. C. 1974.

Guide for Development and Administration of Coordinated Home Care Programs, A. U. S. Department of Health, Education and Welfare. Public Health Service. Publication No. 1579. Division of Medical Care Administration. Superintendent of Documents. U. S. Government Printing Office. Washington, D. C. 1966.

Guide for Promoting Home Health Services, A. U. S. Department of Health, Education and Welfare. Public Health Service. Health Services and Mental Health Administration. Community Health Service. DHEW Publication No. (HSM) 73-6406. Superintendent of Documents. U. S. Government Printing Office. Washington, D. C. Reprinted January, 1973.

Home Care for Persons 55 Years and Over: United States, July 1966-June 1968. U. S. Department of Health, Education and Welfare. National Center for Health Statistics. Publication No. (HSM) 72-1062. Superintendent of Documents. U. S. Government Printing Office. Washington, D. C. 1972.

Home Health Services in the United States. A Report to the Special Committee on Aging. United States Senate. Ninety-second Congress. Second Session. Superintendent of Documents. U. S. Government Printing Office. Washington, D. C. April, 1972.

Krakowski, Martin. Cost-Benefit Analysis of the Foster Grandparent Program. Office of the Assistant Secretary for Planning and Evaluation. U. S. Department of Health, Education and Welfare. Superintendent of Documents. U. S. Government Printing Office. Washington, D. C. 1971.

Leff, Jack. Advocacy in the Field of Aging. Senior Opportunities and Services. Technical Assistance Monograph No. 17. National Council on the Aging. Office of Economic Opportunity. Washington, D. C. October, 1972.

Long, Nicholas, et al. Information and Referral Services: The Resource File. U. S. Department of Health, Education and Welfare. Superintendent of Documents. U. S. Government Printing Office. Washington, D. C. 1973.

Making Services for the Elderly Work: Some Lessons from the British Experience. Special Committee on Aging. United States Senate. Superintendent of Documents. U. S. Government Printing Office. Washington, D. C. November, 1971.

Materials Related to H.R.I.: Aid to Aged, Blind, and Disabled, Social Services, Fiscal Relief for States; July 22, 1971. United States Senate. Finance Committee Ninety-second Congress. First Session. Superintendent of Documents. U. S. Government Printing Office. Washington, D. C. 1971.

Older Americans Comprehensive Services Amendments of 1973. Committee on Labor and Public Welfare. Subcommittee on Aging. United States Senate. Ninety-third Congress. First Session. Superintendent of Documents. U. S. Government Printing Office. Washington, D. C. 1973.

Rogers, Virginia. Guidelines for a Telephone Reassurance Service. Institute of Gerontology. University of Michigan-Wayne State University. Administration on Aging. U. S. Department of Health, Education and Welfare. Superintendent of Documents. U. S. Government Printing Office. Washington, D. C. 1972.

Senior Opportunities and Services. (Directory of Programs). Superintendent of Documents. U. S. Government Printing Office. Washington, D. C. 1975. (Updated annually).

Stough, Ada Barnett. A Rural County Cares for Its Aging. U. S. Department of Health, Education and Welfare. AOA Publication No. 187. Superintendent of Documents. U. S. Government Printing Office. Washington, D. C. Revised. 1967.

Tessari, Diane, et al. Information and Referral Services: Information-Giving and Referral. Administration on Aging. Office of Human Development. U. S. Department of Health, Education and Welfare. DHEW Publication No. (OHD) 75-20112. Superintendent of Documents. U. S. Government Printing Office. Washington, D. C. 1974.

To Find the Way to Opportunities and Services for Older Americans. Administration on Aging. U. S. Department of Health, Education and Welfare. Superintendent of Documents. U. S. Government Printing Office. Washington, D. C. 1975.

To Find the Way to Services in Your Community. Administration on Aging. U. S. Department of Health, Education and Welfare. DHEW Publication No. (SRS) 73-20807. Superintendent of Documents. U. S. Government Printing Office. Washington, D. C. 1973.

Trager, Brahna. Home Health Services in the United States. United States Senate. Special Committee on Aging. Superintendent of Documents. U. S. Government Printing Office. Washington, D. C. 1972.

DEATH AND DYING

Anderson, Dorothy B. and McClean, Lenora J. (Editors). Identifying Suicide Potential. Behavioral Publications, Inc. New York, New York. 1971.

Examination of problems regarding pre-suicidal phenomena. Concrete suggestions are made on how to reach high risk populations and how to spot danger signals in patients.

Bane, J. D., et al (Editors). Death and Ministry; Pastoral Care of the Dying and Bereaved. Seabury Press. New York, New York. 1975.

The multidisciplinary contributors, all of whom are involved in care of the dying and bereaved, have constructed a guide for the clergy.

Brim, Orville G., et al. The Dying Patient. Russell Sage Foundation. New York, New York. 1970.

Collection of articles on problems associated with dying from sociological, economic, medical, and legal points of view.

Browning, Mary H. and Lewis, Edith (Editors). The Dying Patient: A Nursing Perspective. The American Journal of Nursing Company. New York, New York. 1972.

Viewpoints are expressed from various disciplines as well as experiences with dying and bereaved persons; offers material for discussion, study and improvement of professional practice.

Cartwright, Ann, et al. Life Before Death. Routledge and Kegan Paul. Boston, Massachusetts. 1973.

Report by a multidisciplinary team of researchers on both terminally ill patients and their caregivers, and the problems identified. A study made in England but with direct application in the United States.

Cutter, Fred. Coming to Terms with Death. Nelson-Hall, Inc. Chicago, Illinois. 1974.

An examination of contemporary attitudes toward death, with a practical approach to achieving greater dignity and honesty toward the inevitability of death.

Davis, Richard H., and Neiswender, Margaret (Editors). Dealing With Death. The Ethel Percy Andrus Gerontology Center. University of Southern California. Los Angeles, California. 1973.

Proceedings of seminars and workshops on dying. Subjects covered are: the meaning of dying in American society, psychological treatment of the dying patient, suicide among the aged, the practitioner's dilemma, nursing and the dying patient.

Day, Stacey B. Death and Attitudes Toward Death. Proceedings. Bell Museum of Pathology. University of Minnesota Medical School. Minneapolis, Minnesota. 1972.

A symposium on death and attitudes toward death conducted by physicians.

Dempsey, David. The Way We Die. Macmillan Publishing Company. New York, New York. 1975.

A comprehensive account of the experience of dying; the fight against it; accomodation to it; and attempt to transcend it from the viewpoints of the dying and the survivors.

Epstein, Charlotte. Nursing the Dying Patient. Reston Publishing Company. Reston, Virginia. 1975.

A book designed to aid the professional nurse who interacts with dying patients. The seven sections of the book include:

1. Heightening self awareness
2. The stages of dying
3. Trajectories of dying
4. Death at different ages
5. The conspiracy of silence
6. The process of observation
7. Helping the professional

Feldman, Marvin J., et al. Fears Related to Death and Suicide. MSS Information Corporation. New York, New York. 1973.

A discussion of attitudes toward death manifested in dreams and nightmares; psychological theories on death; and attitudes toward death among suicidal subjects.

Focus on Death and Dying. Prepared by the Editorial Staff of "Nursing Digest." Contemporary Publishing, Inc. Wakefield, Massachusetts. 1975.

Topics include: dying in the United States, families in crisis, the dying patient, among others.

Fassler, Joan. _My Grandpa Died Today_. Behavioral Science Publications. New York, New York. 1971.

A simply written book about death for children, sensitive and understanding.

Glaser, Barney and Strauss, Anselm L. _Awareness of Dying_. Aldine Publishing Company. Chicago, Illinois. 1965.

An examination of the dying patient and those about him; provides the basis for a conceptual scheme for understanding reactions to dying.

______________________________. _Time for Dying_. Aldine Publishing Company. Chicago, Illinois. 1968.

Discussion of the reciprocal effect that dying patients, family, staff and institutional structures have upon one another.

Gordon, David Cole. _Overcoming the Fear of Death_. The MacMillan Company. New York, New York. 1970.

A forthright look at man's basic fear of death; draws upon psychological insights derived from both Eastern and Western cultures.

Gorer, Geoffrey. _Death, Grief and Mourning_. Doubleday and Company, Inc. Garden City, New York. 1965.

Analysis of mourning practices and of attitudes toward death in contemporary society based upon interviews with 1,628 people, representing the spectrum of social classes.

Green, Betty R. and Irish, Donald P. (Editors). _Death Education: Preparation for Living_. Proceedings of the Symposium sponsored by Hamline University, St. Paul, Minnesota. Schenkman Publishing Company. Cambridge, Massachusetts. 1971.

Topics include the value of eduation about death and the social, medical and religious connotations of death.

Grief - Its Recognition and Resolution. Gerontology Center. Institute for the Study of Human Development. Pennsylvania State University. University Park, Pennsylvania. 1974.

Proceedings of a national conference held at Pennsylvania State University in November, 1973. A good resource for those interested in basic knowledge on topical subjects in the field of death and dying.

Grollman, Earl A. (Editor). *Concerning Death: A Practical Guide for the Living*. Beacon Press. Boston, Massachusetts. 1974.

A publication which deals with rational and meaningful preparation for death; offers guidelines concerning traumas related to death.

Hinton, John. *Dying*. Penguin Books, Inc. Baltimore, Maryland. 1967.

A review of attitudes toward death, the dying, care of the dying person, and mourning.

Kalish, Richard A., and Reynolds, David K. *Death and Ethnicity: A Psycho-cultural Study*. Ethel Percy Andrus Gerontology Center. University of Southern California. Los Angeles, California. 1976.

Sub-cultural differences in attitudes and reactions to death.

Kastenbaum, Robert J. *Death, Society, and Human Experience*. C. V. Mosby Company. St. Louis, Missouri. 1977.

A textbook that deals with the meaning of death and grief in this society from cultural, historical, psychological, economic and religious perspectives.

____________________, and Aisenberg, Ruth. *The Psychology of Death*. Springer Publishing Company. New York, New York. 1972.

A synthesis of what is known and foreseen about man's changing relationships to death.

Kavanaugh, Robert E. *Facing Death*. Penguin Books, Inc. Baltimore, Maryland. 1974.

A discussion of preconceived notions of mourning, of death mythology and contemporary views of euthanasia, suicide, and the value of funerals in society.

Keleman, Stanley. Living Your Dying. Random House. New York, New York. 1975.

A discussion of the possibilities of changing present attitudes toward death and dying.

Kohl, Marvin (Editor). Beneficent Euthanasia. Prometheus Books. Buffalo, New York. 1975.

The book deals with the subject of euthanasia in relation to social justice and human rights. Subjects covered are religious and ethical issues, dignity, medical and legal issues, suicide and related topics.

Krant, Melvin J. Dying and Dignity: The Meaning and Control of a Personal Death. Charles C. Thomas. Springfield, Illinois. 1974.

A book written primarily for families and the staff who work with dying persons. It attempts to clarify the concept of dignity and meaning as a personal statement in an individual death.

Kübler-Ross, Elisabeth. Death: The Final Stage of Growth. Prentice-Hall, Inc. Englewood Cliffs, New Jersey. 1975.

The author investigates the effects of a society that is death-denying, compares this culture with others, and concludes that growth toward acceptance of mortality for oneself and others gives added meaning to life.

____________________. On Death and Dying: What the Dying Have to Teach Doctors, Nurses, Clergy and Their Own Families. The MacMillan Company. New York, New York. 1969.

Based on interviews with dying patients, this book cites, illustrates and discusses the emotional stages in the process of dying.

____________________. Questions and Answers on Death and Dying. Collier Books. New York, New York. 1974.

A compilation of questions about dying patients and their care frequently posed to the author by professionals and lay audiences together with her answers. Questions are grouped according to topics.

Kutscher, Austin H. (Editor). Death and Bereavement. Charles C. Thomas. Springfield, Illinois. 1969.

Discussion of grief and bereavement with suggestions for working through the processes.

Lester, David. Why People Kill Themselves: A Summary of Research Findings on Suicidal Behavior. Charles C. Thomas. Springfield, Illinois. 1972.

Title self explanatory.

Lofland, Lyn H. Toward a Sociology of Death and Dying. Sage Contemporary Social Science Issues. Beverly Hills, California. 1976.

The author discusses the issues and considers the societal impact of human concerns and technological advances in prolongation of life.

Loss Reaction and Grief Management. Gerontology Center. Institute for the Study of Human Development. Pennsylvania State University. University Park, Pennsylvania. 1976.

A training manual which deals with dying, death and the grief process. Analogies are drawn between death and the role-loss which often occurs in old age.

Mannes, Marya. Last Rights: A Case for the Good Death. New American Library. Bergenfield, New Jersey. 1975.

Religious, philosophical, ethical, and legal aspects are studied, and a plea is made for permitting people the right of deciding how their terminally ill bodies will be treated.

Meyer, Joachim E. Death and Neurosis. (Translated by Margarete Nunberg). International Universities Press, Inc. New York, New York. 1975.

A psychiatrist considers the theory of neuroses in relation to man's mortality, and death in relation to development of neuroses. Not limited to the elderly, attention is given to this population.

Montefiore, Canon H. W., et al. *Death Anxiety: Normal and Pathological Aspects*. MSS Information Corporation. New York, New York. 1973.

A collection of papers which deals with such topics as attitudes toward aging; anxieties related to death, dying, and illness; and some of the ethical problems in the field of geriatrics.

Oaughill, Rita (Editor). *The Dying Patient: A Supportive Approach*. Little, Brown and Company. Boston, Massachusetts. 1976.

Although a majority of the authors are nurses and the major emphasis of the book is medical, some attention also is given to psycho-social aspects.

Ostheimer, Nancy C., and Ostheimer, John M. *Life or Death - Who Controls?* Springer Publishing Company. New York, New York. 1976.

The authors raise social and ethical questions related to modern technological advances in medicine and to individual self control of life.

Parkes, Colin Murray. *Bereavement, Studies of Grief in Adult Life*. International Universities Press, Inc. New York, New York. 1972.

Discussion of bereavement and its physical and mental consequences; offers approaches to helping the bereaved.

Pearson, Leonard (Editor). *Death and Dying: Current Issues in the Treatment of the Dying Person*. The Press of Case Western Reserve University. Cleveland, Ohio. 1969.

In addition to dealing with treatment of terminally ill patients, the book also includes a section devoted to families of dying patients.

Pincus, Lily. *Death and the Family: The Importance of Mourning*. Vintage Books-Random House. New York, New York. 1976.

Emphasis is given to the therapeutic value of mourning and the social customs which support it.

Pine, Vanderlyn R., et al (Editors). Acute Grief and the Funeral. Charles C. Thomas. Springfield, Illinois. 1976.

A collection of papers dealing with the psychological and social ramifications of grief and bereavement.

Russell, Ruth O. Freedom to Die: Moral and Legal Aspects of Euthanasia. Human Sciences Press. Behavioral Publications, Inc. New York, New York. 1975.

A book which questions whether old ethical, religious, and legal standards are appropriate for the new medical technology.

Schnaper, Nathan, et al. Management of the Dying Patient and His Family. MSS Information Corporation. New York, New York. 1973.

Emphasis is upon fears and reactions of the dying patient and of his family; emotional factors in professional service personnel responses to the terminally ill patient. Problems of patient isolation and moral responsibilities also are included.

Schneidman, Edwin S. (Editor). Death: Current Perspectives. Mayfield. Palo Alto, California. 1976.

A compilation of papers which taken together represent the spectrum of views on death and dying.

__________________. Deaths of Man. Penguin Books, Inc. Baltimore, Maryland. 1974.

An examination of death, emphasizing the dying person and his survivors rather than clinical care.

__________________ (Editor). On the Nature of Suicide. Jossey-Bass, Inc. San Francisco, California. 1969.

A collection of papers representing a variety of views and beliefs about suicide.

Schoenberg, Bernard, et al (Editors). Anticipatory Grief. Columbia University Press. New York, New York. 1974.

A multidisciplinary approach to the understanding of grief; includes an examination of methods of intervention in the best interests of patient, family, and care givers.

Schoenberg, Bernard, et al (Editors). Bereavement: Its Psychosocial Aspects. Columbia University Press. New York, New York. 1975.

A new collection from the Foundation of Thanatology, which offers techniques for effective intervention in meeting the needs of the bereaved; especially oriented to those in the health field.

__________________. Loss and Grief: Psychological Management in Medical Practice. Columbia University Press. New York, New York. 1970.

Identification of concepts and practices in care of the terminally ill; deals with loss of biological function and with the psychological aspects of death for both patients and family.

Scott, Frances G. and Brewer, Ruth M. (Editors). Confrontations of Death: A Book of Readings and A Suggested Method of Instruction. Oregon Center for Gerontology. Corvallis, Oregon. 1971.

Essays on death and dying which focus upon personal death and feelings toward dying, aging and the aged.

Shibles, Warren. Death: An Interdisciplinary Analysis. Language Press. Whitewater, Wisconsin. 1974.

A scholarly work on death which ranges from Biblical references to Shakespeare and to modern funeral directors. Thoughtful and provocative.

Spark, Muriel. Memento Mori. Aven Books. New York, New York. 1973.

A discussion of habits, ways of life and attitudes toward dying held by older people.

Sudnow, David. Passing On: The Social Organization of Dying. Prentice-Hall, Inc. Englewood Cliffs, New Jersey. 1967.

A sociologist offers his description of the social organization of those whose daily occupations involve caring for the dead and the dying.

Troup, Stanley B., and Grune, William (Editors). *The Patient, Death and the Family*. Charles Scribner's Sons. New York, New York. 1974.

Coverage is concerned with the physician's feelings about a dying patient and his relationship with the family. Includes child as well as adult. Personal experiences are included.

Veatch, Robert M. *Death and Dying*. Claretian Publications. Chicago, Illinois. 1971.

Discussion of the ethical, medical and religious issues surrounding death; emphasis on care of the dying person.

________________. *Death, Dying and the Biological Revolution: Our Last Quest for Responsibility*. Yale University Press. New Haven, Connecticut. 1976.

The author considers public policy issues associated with current "right to die" demands, and gives an analysis of the court cases which have developed.

Vernon, Glenn M. *Sociology of Death: An Analysis of Death Related Behavior*. Ronald Press. New York, New York. 1970.

Consideration of living arrangements and the mental and physical conditions of aging parents. Concrete actions are suggested.

Verwoerdt, Adriaan (Editor). *Communications With the Fatally Ill*. Charles C. Thomas. Springfield, Illinois. 1966.

Contents cover a range of considerations, including the meaning of fatal illness, communications, emotional reactions and their management, family, religious and ethnic aspects, euthanasia.

Watson, Wilbur H., and Maxwell, Robert J. *Human Aging and Dying: A Study in Sociocultural Gerontology*. St. Martin's Press. New York, New York. 1977.

A sociocultural perspective on the processes of aging and dying with reference to twenty-six different societies.

Weatherhead, Leslie D. *Life Begins at Death*. Abingdon Press. Nashville, Tennessee. 1969.

A religious orientation to death.

Weisman, Avery D. On Dying and Denying: A Psychiatric Study of Terminality. Behavioral Publications. New York, New York. 1972.

The relationship between critical, life threatening illness and denial reactions; offers guidance for achieving death with dignity.

________________ and Kastenbaum, Robert. The Psychological Autopsy. Behavioral Publications, Inc. New York, New York. 1968.

Synthesis of medical, social and psychiatric information together with suggested techniques for improving care to the dying patient.

Wilson, Jerry B. Death By Decision: The Medical, Moral and Legal Dilemmas of Euthanasia. Westminster Press. Philadelphia, Pennsylvania. 1975.

A book dealing with the complex issues surrounding terminal care of the ill and the practice of euthanasia.

U. S. GOVERNMENT PUBLICATIONS

Death With Dignity: An Inquiry into Related Public Issues. Special Committee on Aging. United States Senate. Ninety-Second Congress. Second Session. Superintendent of Documents. U. S. Government Printing Office. Washington, D. C. 1972.

Vernick, Joel J. Death and Dying: A Selected Bibliography. U. S. Government Printing Office. Washington, D. C. 1970.

DEMOGRAPHIC DATA

Barsby, S. L., and Cox, D. R. *Interstate Migration of the Elderly: An Economic Analysis*. D. C. Heath & Company. Lexington, Massachusetts. 1975.

Report of a study of factors affecting interstate migration rates of older adults.

Brotman, Herman B. *Who Are the Aged: A Demographic View*. Occasional Papers in Gerontology. Institute of Gerontology. University of Michigan. Ann Arbor, Michigan. 1968.

A concise demographic review of America's older population in the late sixties.

Elderly in America, The: Population Bulletin. Vol. 30, No. 3. Population Reference Bureau, Inc. Washington, D. C. 1975.

A small book of statistics, definitions, and forecasts concerning the aged in the United States.

Fact Book on Aging. National Council on the Aging, Inc. Washington, D. C. 1976.

Data on the aged population characteristics in relation to housing, health, employment, safety, education, family, veterans.

Honnen, James S., et al. *Retirement and Migration in the North-Central States; Comparative Socio-economic Analysis-Wisconsin and Florida*. (Population Series No. 19). Department of Rural Sociology. College of Agriculture and Life Sciences. University of Wisconsin. Madison, Wisconsin. 1969.

Study of 537 respondents and their socio-economic characteristics, migration patterns, age at retirement, marital status and family pattern, educational attainment, income, health, and retirement decision making.

Impact of Middle-Aged and Older Persons in the Population and in the Labor Force (Facts and Trends No. 2). National Council on the Aging, Inc. Washington, D.C. 1973.

Title self-explanatory.

Niebanck, Paul L. and Pope, John B. *The Elderly in Older Urban Areas: Problems of Adaptation and the Effects of Relocation.* Institute for Environmental Studies. University of Pennsylvania. Philadelphia, Pennsylvania. 1965.

A report of the various aspects of relocation of the elderly, including personal ramifications, as well as the impact upon the community.

Palmore, Erdman and Jeffers, Frances C. (Editors) *Prediction of Life Span.* D. C. Heath and Company. Lexington, Massachusetts. 1974.

Predictors of longevity are explored as well as how to sustain a better life quality throughout the entire life span.

U.S. GOVERNMENT PUBLICATIONS

Age and Earnings by Occupation for United States, 1970. Census Bureau. U.S. Department of Commerce. Superintendent of Documents. U.S. Government Printing Office. Washington, D.C. 1973.

Age of Population of United States, 1970. Census Bureau. U.S. Department of Commerce. Superintendent of Documents. U.S. Government Printing Office. Washington, D.C. 1972.

Boxby, Lenore,E., et al. *Demographic and Economic Characteristics of the Aged: 1968 Social Security Survey.* U.S. Department of Health, Education, and Welfare. Social Security Administration, Office of Research and Statistics. U.S. Government Printing Office. Washington, D.C. 1975.

Brotman, Herman B. and Williams, Blanch S. _Facts and Figures on Older Americans: State Trends 1950-70_. Administration on Aging. U.S. Department of Health, Education, and Welfare. DHEW Publication No. (SRS) 73-20007. Superintendent of Documents. U.S. Government Printing Office. Washington, D.C. 1973.

Characteristics of the Low-Income Population, 1970. Current Population Reports, Series P-60, No. 81. U.S. Bureau of the Census. Superintendent of Documents. U.S. Government Printing Office. Washington, D.C. 1971.

Current Population Reports; Population Characteristics. Series P-20, No. 279 (March, 1975) "Population Profile of the United States, 1974." U.S. Government Printing Office. Washington, D.C.

Facts and Figures on Older Americans No. 9. The Older American Indian Population: Geographic Distribution 1970. U.S. Department of Health, Education, and Welfare. Administration on Aging. Superintendent of Documents. U.S. Government Printing Office. Washington, D.C. 1974.

Mobility of the Population of the United States: March 1970 to March 1975. Current Population Reports, Series P-20, No. 285. U.S. Bureau of Census. Washington, D.C. 1975.

New Facts About Older Americans. Office of Human Development. Administration on Aging. U.S. Department of Health, Education, and Welfare. DHEW Publication No. (SRS) 73-20006. Superintendent of Documents. U.S. Government Printing Office. Washington, D.C. 1973.

Population, Housing and Income and Federal Housing Programs. U.S. Department of Housing and Urban Development. Superintendent of Documents. U.S. Government Printing Office. Washington, D.C. 1971.

Projections of Population of Voting Age for States. Census Bureau. U.S. Department of Commerce. Superintendent of Documents. U.S. Government Printing Office. Washington, D.C. 1972.

Seraile, Elmore J. Social and Economic Characteristics of the Older Population, 1974. Population Division. Census Bureau. U. S. Department of Commerce. Suitland, Maryland. 1975.

Siegel, Jacob S., et al. Demographic Aspects of Aging and the Older Population in the United States. U. S. Bureau of the Census. Current Population Report, Series P-23. No. 59. U. S. Government Printing Office. Washington, D. C. 1976.

Veteran Age 65 and Over: A Profile, The. U. S. Veterans Administration. Washington, D. C. 1968.

DENTAL AND ORAL HEALTH

Davidoff, Arthur, et al (Editors). Dentistry for the special Patient: The Aged, Chronically Ill and Handicapped. W. B. Saunders Company. Philadelphia, Pennsylvania. 1972.

A guide to which twenty-five specialists have contributed background information and management techniques designed to overcome problems of dental care for geriatric patients, and for those handicapped as a result of stroke, cerebral palsy and other disabling diseases.

Easlick, Kenneth A. (Editor). Proceedings of the Workshop on Community Action to Promote the Oral Health of the Chronically Ill, Handicapped and the Aged. School of Public Health. The University of Michigan. Ann Arbor, Michigan. 1965.

This workshop report includes a survey of the oral health needs of the chronically ill and aged, an explanation of community actions programs, and suggestion for initiating and coordinating community programs.

Franks, A. S. T. and Hedgegard, Björn. Geriatric Dentistry. F. A. Davis Company. Philadelphia, Pennsylvania. 1973.

This book deals with the basis for understanding oral and facial disorders in the elderly, their context, background and treatment. Students, dental professionsals and associated professions interested in human aging problems will find this book a helpful resource.

Kutscher, Austin H. and Goldberg, Ivan K. (Editors). Oral Care of the Aging and Dying Patient. Charles C. Thomas. Springfield, Illinois. 1973.

Examination of the ethical and practical considerations of when, what, and how to treat the special problems of the elderly and the dying patient; a discussion of oral conditions and disease entities specific to these patients.

Waldman, H. Barry and Stein, Murray. A Plan for Total Dental Services for the Chronically Ill and Aged. Highland View Hospital Department of Dentistry. Cleveland, Ohio. 1967.

Description of a home care and outpatient dental program for the aged and seriously disabled.

U.S. GOVERNMENT PUBLICATIONS

Portraits in Community Health: Dental Care for the Chronically Ill. U.S. Public Health Service. Publication No. 1344. Superintendent of Documents. U.S. Government Printing Office. Washington, D.C. 1967.

DISEASES AND DISABILITIES

Adams, J. Crawford. Arthritis and Back Pain. University Park Press. Baltimore, Maryland. 1972.

Written for professional health care personnel, this book offers practical, medical information which can be helpful also to arthritis patients and to other professional service personnel concerned with social aspects of the disease.

Berezin, Martin A., and Cath, Stanley H. (Editors). Geriatric Psychiatry: Loss and Emotional Disorders in the Aging Process. International Universities Press. New York, New York. 1967.

A collection of papers presented at symposia arranged by the Boston Society for Gerontologic Psychiatry; covers psychiatric disorders associated with old age.

Bloom, Arnold. Diabetes Explained. University Park Press. Baltimore, Maryland. 1971.

This book covers symptoms, diagnosis, complications, treatment and care of the person with diabetes, a disease prevalent among older persons.

Gardner, Dugald Lindsay. The Pathology of Rheumatoid Arthritis. Williams and Wilkins. Baltimore, Maryland. 1972.

A guide for pathologists, physicians and surgeons concerned with rheumatic and connective tissue diseases.

Goldfarb, Alvin I. Aging and Organic Brain Syndrome. Health Learning Systems, Inc. Bloomfield, New Jersey. 1974.

A description of conditions categorized as organic brain syndrome with emphasis upon recognizing types involved and treatment available.

Harris, Luke. Geriatric Chest Disease. John Wright and Sons, Ltd./ Williams and Wilkins. Baltimore, Maryland. 1974.

Title self explanatory.

Hauss, W. H., and Oberwittler (Editors). Geriatrie in der Praxis. Springer Verlag. Berlin, Germany. New York, New York. 1975.

Although this volume begins with psychological and social aspects of aging and a section on homes for the aged, major attention is devoted to diseases more prevalent in later life. Included also are: nutrition, exercise and other topics.

Healey, Louis A., et al. Beyond the Copper Bracelet. Charles C. Thomas. Springfield, Illinois. 1972.

Myths and facts on arthritis.

Jayson, Malcolm I. V. and Dixon, Allan St. J. Understanding Arthritis and Rheumatism: A Complete Guide to the Problems and Treatments. Pantheon Books. New York, New York. 1974.

A detailed discussion of the causes, problems, and treatment of arthritis and rheumatism.

Lowenthal, Marjorie Fiske and Berkman,Paul L. Aging and Mental Disorders in San Francisco: A Social Psychiatric Study. Jossey-Bass, Inc. San Francisco, California. 1967.

A comparative study of institutionalized and non-institutionalized people over 60 years of age suffering from similar mental disorders.

McCarron, Margaret M. and McCormick,Ruth A. Acute Organic Disorder Accompanied by Mental Symptons: Recognizing Treatable Physiological Causes of Acute Brain Syndrome. Office of Planning. California Department of Mental Hygiene. Sacramento, California. 1967.

Title self explanatory.

McKeown, Florence. Pathology of the Aged. Butterworth. London, England. 1965.

Focus is primarily on malignancy and diseases of the heart and nervous system.

Myers, Julian S. (Editor). An Orientation to Chronic Disease and Disability. The Macmillan Company. New York, New York. 1965.

A survey of chronic diseases covering the systems of the body.

Post, Felix. Persistent Persecutory States of the Elderly. Pergamon Press Publishing Company. New York, New York. 1966.

A review of the literature on late-life schizophrenia and a summary of 100 case histories of elderly patients with this disability.

Riklan, Manuel. L-Dopa and Parkinsonism: A Psychological Assessment. Charles C. Thomas. Springfield, Illinois. 1973.

Title self explanatory; discusses both positive and negative behavioral effects.

Schwartz, Arthur N. Etiology of Mental Disorders in Aging. The Ethel Percy Andrus Gerontology Center. University of Southern California. Los Angeles, California. 1975.

A bibliography.

Services for Elderly Deaf Persons: Recommended Policies and Programs. Deafness Research and Training Center. New York University. New York, New York. 1971.

A summary of comprehensive recommendations for action on behalf of elderly deaf people, proposed at a conference of leaders in this field. Recommendations were adopted by the White House Conference on Aging.

Sokoloff, Leon. The Biology of Degenerative Joint Disease. The University of Chicago Press. Chicago, Illinois. 1969.

A systematic treatise on the pathogenesis of degenerative joint disease. Topics include history, morphology, pathology, comparative pathology, biochemistry, repair, and biomechanics. It offers a basis for research, and points out needs for further study.

Taylor, Robert B. Feeling Alive After 65. Arlington House. New Rochelle, New York. 1973.

A discussion of organ deterioration associated with the aging process; also includes advice on diet, retirement, sexual activity, etc.

Thomas, J. H. Blood Disorders in the Elderly. John Wright and Sons, Ltd./Williams and Wilkins. Baltimore, Maryland. 1971.

Title self explanatory.

Ullman, Montague. Behavioral Changes in Patients Following Strokes. Charles C. Thomas. Springfield, Illinois. 1962.

Exerpts from case histories illustrating the span of mood changes in psychological reactions during acute and chronic phases of vascular disease. An old book which offers information still current.

Verbov, Julian. Skin Diseases in the Elderly. J. B. Lippincott Company. Philadelphia, Pennsylvania. 1975.

The audience for this British book on clinical geriatric dermatology is primarily dermatology residents. However, it offers a concise reference for general practitioners and other medical students, especially in the area of skin conditions symptomatic of systemic disorders.

Walford, Roy L. The Immunologic Theory of Aging. Williams and Wilkins. Baltimore, Maryland. 1970.

Discussion of auto-immunity and its role in the aging process.

______________, et al. The Relation of Aging to Immunity. MSS Information Corporation. New York, New York. 1973.

This book considers the immunological effects of aging with respect to disease states, malignancies, autoimmunity, and immunologic tolerance.

Wolstenholme, G. E. W. and O'Connor, Maeve. (Editors). Alzheimer's Disease and Related Conditions: A Ciba Foundation Symposium. J. A. Churchill. London, England. 1970.

Causes of age-linked mental deficits and the relationships between biological and pathological aging are the two important issues discussed in this volume.

U.S. GOVERNMENT PUBLICATIONS

Arteriosclerosis: Report by National Heart and Lung Institute Task Force on Arteriosclerosis. Volumes I and II. U.S. Department of Health, Education, and Welfare. National Institutes of Health. DHEW Publication No. (NIH) 72-219. Superintendent of Documents. U.S. Government Printing Office. Washington, D.C. June, 1971.

Hardening of the Arteries: Cause of Heart Attacks. U.S. Department of Health, Education, and Welfare. Public Health Service. National Institutes of Health. DHEW Publication No. (NIH) 72-251. Superintendent of Documents. U.S. Government Printing Office. Washington, D.C. Reprinted 1972.

Mental Disorders of Aging. U.S. Department of Health, Education, and Welfare. Public Health Service. Reprint. Superintendent of Documents. U.S. Government Printing Office. Washington, D.C. 1967.

Ostfeld, Adrian M. and Gibson, Don C. (Editors). Epidemiology of Aging. U.S. Department of Health, Education, and Welfare. Public Health Service. DHEW Publication No. (NIH) 75-711. Superintendent of Documents. U.S. Government Printing Office. Washington, D.C. 1975.

DRUGS AND THE AGED

Buerki, Robert A. (Editor). Pharmaceutical Services for Nursing Homes. Ohio State University. Columbus, Ohio. 1966.

State and Federal provisions for pharmaceutical services to nursing home patients.

Davis, Richard H., and Smith, William K. (Editors). Drugs and the Elderly. Ethel Percy Andrus Gerontology Center. University of Southern California. Los Angeles, California. 1973.

Discussion of the benefits derived from drug therapies for the elderly, and the problems associated with misuse of drugs. Topics range from drug interaction to self medication.

Eisdorfer, Carl, and Fann, William E. (Editors). Psychopharmacology and Aging. Plenum Publishing Corporation. New York, New York. 1973.

An examination of clinical uses and effects of psycho-active agents upon the physical and mental conditions of aged patients. Reports research findings as well as abuse potentials, patient management, and health care facility use of drugs.

Fann, William E., and Maddox, George L. (Editors). Drug Issues in Geropsychiatry. Williams and Wilkins Company. Baltimore, Maryland. 1974.

These proceedings of a conference held at Duke University combine emphases upon 1) problems related to aging; 2) use of drugs with the aged and related problems; and 3) patient and professional staff interactions related to drug management.

Freeman, Joseph T. (Editor). Clinical Principles and Drugs in the Aging. Charles C. Thomas. Springfield, Illinois. 1963.

Pertinent facts and principles in the use of drugs with older patients; twenty-six clinicians and pharmacologists cover various subjects.

Pharmaceutical Services in the Long Term Facility. Seventh Edition. American Health Care Association. American Pharmaceutical Association and American Society of Hospital Pharmacists. American Pharmaceutical Association. Washington. D.C. 1975.

A guide not only for pharmaceutical services, but also for classification of drugs designed to assist professional staff. Included also is pertinent information on regulatory controls, selected references and an evaluation guide.

"Psychopharmacology In the Aged." Journal of Geriatric Psychiatry. Vol. 7. 1974.

A collection of papers read at the 13th Annual Scientific Meeting of the Boston Society for Gerontologic Psychiatry.

ECONOMICS OF AGING

Adler, Joan. The Retirement Book: A Complete Early Planning Guide to Finances, New Activities, and Where to Live. William Morrow and Company, Inc. New York, New York. 1975.

This source discusses the financial aspects of the retirement years and stresses the importance of careful and thoughtful planning.

Barfield, Richard E. and Morgan, James N. Early Retirement: The Decision and the Experience and the Automobile Worker and Retirement: A Second Look. Institute for Social Research. University of Michigan. Ann Arbor, Michigan. 1974.

The first part of this book reports a study of the pension plan of the United Automobile Workers first published in 1969. The second part is a follow-up survey of workers and pensioners included in the original study.

Bleakney, T. P. Retirement Systems for Public Employees. Richard D. Irwin. Homewood, Illinois. 1972.

A book designed to further the understanding of public employee retirement systems by legislators and others responsible for their functioning.

Bowen, William G., et al. (Editors). The Princeton Symposium On the American System of Social Insurance; Its Philosophy, Impact, and Future Development. McGraw-Hill. New York, New York. 1968.

Much of this material is related to the provision of income to the aged.

Brennan, Michael J., et al. The Economics of Age. W. W. Norton and Company. New York, New York. 1967.

A study of economic forces that determine income and employment at different age levels. Emphasis is upon problems that confront older workers.

Brinker, Paul A. Economic Insecurity and Social Security. Appleton-Century-Crofts. New York, New York. 1968

A review of perspectives, problems, and solutions related to public assistance programs serving the aged, disabled, and low-income persons.

Bryden, Kenneth. Old Age Pensions and Policy-Making in Canada. McGill-Queen's University Press. Montreal, Canada. 1974.

A case study of old age pensions in Canada and the politics involved in income redistribution.

Consumer Training Guide for the Elderly. Office of Consumer Affairs and the Office of Aging. Georgia Department of Human Resources. 50 Seventh Street, N. E. Atlanta, Georgia 30323.

A handbook resulting from the research completed by VISTA volunteers which offers practical information on prescription drugs, health insurance, Medicaid and Medicare, non-prescription drugs and devices, mail order health insurance, and drug plans and discount clubs.

Ducovny, Amram. The Billion $ Swindle: Frauds Against the Elderly. Fleet Press. New York, New York. 1969.

An expose of fraud in the areas of health and nutrition, medicine, finance, and funerals.

Early Retirement: A Survey of Company Policies and Retirees' Experiences. College of Business Administration. University of Oregon. Eugene, Oregon. 1969.

Report on a study designed to delineate policies and pension plan options, and to assess how retirees had fared economically under the plans.

Economics of Aging: Toward 2001, The Institute of Gerontology. University of Michigan. Ann Arbor, Michigan. 1976.

The proceedings of a 1975 Conference concerned with projected economic needs of the aged in the United States and alternatives for meeting them.

Ford, Norman D. Increasing Your Retirement and Other Income. Fifth Edition. Harian Publications. New York, New York. 1968.

Sources of second income are discussed.

Future of Aging and the Aged, The. Southern Newspaper Publishers Association Foundations. Atlanta, Georgia. 1971.

This book is concerned with the economics of aging and necessary adaptations. Includes extensive supporting statistical evidence.

Greenough, William C., and King, Francis P. Pension Plans and Public Policy. Columbia University Press. Irvington-on-Hudson, New York. 1976.

An authoritative and comprehensive examination of the development of public and private pension plans in both the United States and Western Europe during the past century, and of present sources, types and extent of retirement incomes.

Guide to Income Maintenance and Other Legal Problems of Older Adults. Legal Aid Society. Cincinnati, Ohio. 1975.

A handbook designed to serve as a guide in the area of income maintenance, rather than a detailed coverage of the subject. It is a nontechnical manual including a variety of topics.

Heidbreder, Elizabeth M. Retirement Income: A Selected Bibliography of Facts, Issues, and Practical Information. National Council on the Aging. Washington, D. C. 1972.

An annotated bibliography including books, articles and government publications on budgets, social security and public and private pensions.

Ingraham, Mark H., and Mulanaphy, James M. My Purpose Holds. Teachers Insurance and Annuity Association of America. New York, New York. 1974.

A report based upon a study of 2269 annuitants under TIAA and College Retirement Equities Fund. Respondents evaluated the adequacy of their incomes.

Katona, George. Private Pensions and Individual Savings. Survey Research Center. Institute for Social Research. University of Michigan. Ann Arbor, Michigan. 1965.

Analysis of the economic behavior of persons covered by pension plans.

Kreps, Juanita M. Lifetime Allocation of Work and Income: Essays in the Economics of Aging. Duke University Press. Durham, North Carolina. 1971.

A book covering the broad questions of work and income; discusses the mechanism of timing of work. Attention is directed to recent developments in work and earnings during the life span.

Life Insurances Fact Book for 1976. American Council of Life Insurance. 277 Park Avenue. New York, New York. 1976.

The 31st edition of a compilation of charts, tables and other information which provides extensive data about insurance related to middle-aged and older American families.

List of Worthwhile Life and Health Insurance Books, A. Institute of Life Insurance and Health Insurance Institute. New York, New York. 1970.

A comprehensive resource guide on personal insurance.

Lurie, Irene. Integrating Income Maintenance Programs. Academic Press. New York, New York. 1975.

One of the monograph series of the Institute for Research and Poverty, University of Wisconsin. The purpose of this investigation was to determine the extent of integration among the several Federal income maintenance programs. The audience for whom this was written is economists.

Margolius, Sidney. Your Personal Guide to Successful Retirement. Random House. New York, New York. 1969.

A handbook on retirement with specific emphasis given to the financial aspects.

Margolius, Sidney, et al. The Aging Consumer. Occasional Papers in Gerontology. Institute of Gerontology. University of Michigan. Ann Arbor, Michigan. 1972.

An examination of older persons coping with inflation and the complexities of the market place. Demonstrates the need for government protection.

Nader, Ralph and Blackwell, Kate. You and Your Pension. Grossman Publishers. New York, New York. 1973.

Written for the millions who expect pensions but never receive them, this book lists the shortcomings of the private pension plans which so many people depend upon for retirement income.

Pension Facts - 1975. Institute of Life Insurance. New York, New York. 1976.

An annual publication designed as a reference. Reviews the history of pensions in the United States, reports on legislative provisions, and gives a bibliography of literature in this field.

Pension Reform Act of 1974: P.L. 93-406. Commerce Clearing House. New York, New York. 1974.

Publication includes the Act and an explanation of it as well as Committee reports.

Peterson, David A. The Crisis in Retirement Finance: The Perceptions of Older Americans. Occasional Papers in Gerontology. Institute of Gerontology. University of Michigan. Ann Arbor, Michigan. 1972.

An investigation of attitudes of older people toward government income maintenance policies. Suggestions are included for policy changes and political action among the aged.

Pilch, Michael and Wood, Victor. Pension Scheme Practice. Hutchinson Press. London, England. 1967.

Publication offering the layman some factual guidance on pension practices.

Private Pensions and the Public Interest: A Symposium Sponsored by American Enterprise Institute for Public Policy Research. American Enterprise Institute for Public Policy Research. Washington, D. C. 1970.

Evaluation and analysis of public and private pension systems and their practices.

Retirement Income. The National Council on the Aging, Inc. Washington, D. C. Revised periodically.

An annotated bibliography.

Retirement Planning Leadership Conference. Institute of Life Insurance. New York, New York. 1970.

A conference held by the Institute of Life Insurance to examine the role and opportunities of life insurance companies in retirement planning. Those attending included insurance personnel, group pension clients and specialists in the aging field.

Rohrlich, George F.(Editor). Social Economics for the 1970's: Programs for Social Security, Health and Manpower. Dunellen. New York, New York. 1970.

An overview of problems and proposed solutions to socioeconomic conditions in the United States, which includes the social security system, health care, income maintenance, and public welfare.

Schmid, W. Williams. Retirement Systems of the American Teacher. Fleet Press. New York, New York. 1970.

Title is self explanatory.

Schulz, James H. The Economics of Aging. Wadsworth Publishing Company. Belmont, California. 1976.

A synthesis of the current economic status of the aging and the socio-economic issues surrounding this topic.

Schulz, James, et al. Providing Adequate Retirement Income. University Press of New England. Hanover, New Hampshire. 1975.

An examination of the current economic status of the elderly in the U. S., with projections of future retirement income and consideration of alternative policies concerning income. In addition to the U. S., old age pension reforms in four other countries are surveyed, e.g., Sweden, the Federal Republic of Germany, Belgium, and Canada.

State and Local Employee Pension Systems. Tax Foundation. New York, New York. 1969.

An examination of state and local government pension systems pointing out problems; offers appraisal of future developments.

Study of Corporate Pension Plans. Bankers Trust Company. The Bankers Trust Company. New York, New York. 1975.

Report of a study of current practices in corporate pension plans in large United States corporations; summarizes changes in plans between 1970 and 1975; and gives the results of cooperative findings for a previous study. This is the tenth report of a series of studies of pension plans between 1943 and 1975.

Study of Industrial Retirement Plans. Bankers Trust. New York, New York. 1970.

Analysis of established pension plans adopted between the years 1965 through 1970.

Swartz, Melvin Jay. Don't Die Broke! A Guide to Secure Retirement. Macmillan Publishing Company, Inc. New York, New York. 1975.

Written by an attorney who has served as legal counsel for many retired persons, the book covers pre-retirement planning, and legal and financial matters that must be handled after retirement. Written clearly and understandably in lay language.

Tax Facts for Older Americans: A Comparative Guide to State Tax Regulations. National Retired Teachers Association. American Association of Retired Persons. Washington, D. C. Published annually.

A broad overview of the tax structure in each of the 50 states from the standpoint of regulations of concern to retired taxpayers.

Tilove, Robert. Public Employee Pension Funds. Columbia University Press. New York, New York. 1976.

A Twentieth Century Fund report, this publication covers both Federal and state civil service pension funds and those for local government employees.

Tucker, James F. Current Economic Issues and Problems. Rand McNally College Publishing Company. Chicago, Illinois. 1976.

One chapter deals with distribution of wealth and with social security as a system for redistribution of wealth. Another deals with Medicare and Medicaid and their effects upon health care costs.

U.S. GOVERNMENT PUBLICATIONS

Characteristics of State Public Assistance Plans Under Social Security Act: Old-Age Assistance to Blind, Aid to Families with Dependent Children, Aid to Permanently and Totally Disabled, Aid to Aged, Blind, or Disabled, General Provisions-Eligibility, Assistance, Administration. Division of Program Implementation and Review. Social and Rehabilitation Service, U.S. Department of Health, Education, and Welfare. DHEW Publication No. (SRS) 74-21215. Superintendent of Documents. U.S. Government Printing Office. Washington, D.C. 1973.

Chen, Yung-Ping. Income: Background and Issues. Prepared for the White House Conference on Aging. Superintendent of Documents. U.S. Government Printing Office. Washington, D.C. 1971.

Cruikshank, Nelson H. The Stake of Todays' Workers in Retirement Security: A Working Paper in Conjunction With the Overall Study of "Economics of Aging: Toward a Full Share in Abundance." Special Committee on Aging. United States Senate. Ninety-First Congress. Second Session. Superintendent of Documents. U.S. Government Printing Office. Washington, D.C. 1970.

Digest of 100 Selected Pension Plans Under Collective Bargaining. U. S. Bureau of Labor Statistics. Bulletin No. 1597. Superintendent of Documents. U. S. Government Printing Office. Washington, D. C. 1968.

Dignity Instead of Desperation. Economic Opportunity Office. Executive Office of the President. Superintendent of Documents. U. S. Government Printing Office. Washington, D. C. 1972.

Economic Problems of Aging Women. Hearing before the Subcommittee on Retirement Income and Employment of the House Select Committee on Aging, July 15, 1975. Ninety-fourth Congress. First Session. Superintendent of Documents. U. S. Government Printing Office. Washington, D. C. 1975

Economics of Aging: Toward A Full Share of Abundance. Senate Special Committee on Aging. Ninety-first Congress. Second Session. Report No. 91-1548. Superintendent of Documents. U. S. Government Printing Office. Washington, D. C. 1970.

Employment Aspects of the Economics of Aging: A Working Paper in Conjunction with the Overall Study of Economics of Aging; Toward A Full Share in Abundance. National Institute of Industrial Gerontology. Ninety-first Congress. First Session. Superintendent of Documents. U. S. Government Printing Office. Washington, D. C. 1969.

Federal Benefits for Veterans and Dependents. The Veterans Administration. Available from VA Offices or from Superintendent of Documents. U. S. Government Printing Office. Washington, D. C. 1977. (Revised periodically).

Grad, Susan. _Relative Importance of Income Sources of Aged._ Social Security Administration. U. S. Department of Health, Education and Welfare. DHEW Publication No. (SSA) 73-10033. Superintendent of Documents. U. S. Government Printing Office. Washington, D. C. 1973.

Health Aspects of the Economics of Aging: A Working Paper in Conjunction With the Overall Study of "Economics of Aging: Toward A Full Share of Abundance." Special Committee on Aging. United States Senate. Ninety-first Congress. First Session. Superintendent of Documents. U. S. Government Printing office. Washington, D. C. Revised 1969.

Impact of Rising Energy Costs on Older Americans, The. Hearings before the Senate Special Committee on Aging. U. S. Senate. Superintendent of Documents. U. S. Government Printing Office. Washington, D. C. 1975.

Impact of the Tax Structure on the Elderly, The. The Federal Council on the Aging. U. S. Department of Health, Education and Welfare. National Clearinghouse on the Aging. Washington, D. C. 1976.

Income Security for Older Women: Path to Equality. Subcommittee on Retirement. House Select Committee on Aging. Ninety-fourth Congress. Superintendent of Documents. U. S. Government Printing Office. Washington, D. C. 1975.

Old Age Income Assurance: A Compendium of Papers on Problems and Policy Issues in the Public and Private Pension System. Joint Economic Committee. United States Congress. Ninetieth Congress. First Session. Superintendent of Documents. U.S. Government Printing Office. Washington, D.C. 1967.

Pension Aspects of the Economics of Aging: Present and Future Roles of Private Pensions. Special Committee on Aging. United States Senate. Ninety-First Congress. Second Session. Superintendent of Documents. U.S. Government Printing Office. Washington, D.C. 1970.

Poverty Amid Plenty, The American Paradox: Report. U.S. President's Commission on Income Maintenance Programs. Superintendent of Documents. U.S. Government Printing Office. Washington, D.C. 1969.

Private Pension Plan Benefits. U.S. Bureau of Labor Statistics. Bulletin No. 1485. Superintendent of Documents. U.S. Government Printing Office. Washington, D.C. 1966.

Proposed Fiscal 1977 Budget: What It Means for Older Americans. Special Committee on Aging. Ninety-Fourth Congress. Second Session. U.S. Senate. Superintendent of Documents. U.S. Government Printing Office. Washington, D.C. 1976. Updated annually.

Proposed USDA Food Stamp Cutbacks For the Elderly. Hearing Before the Special Committee on Aging. United States Senate. Ninety-Fourth Congress. First Session. November 3, 1975. Superintendent of Documents. U.S. Government Printing Office. Washington, D.C. 1976.

Protecting Older Americans Against Overpayment of Income Taxes (A Checklist of Itemized Deductions). Prepared by the Special Committee on Aging. United States Senate. Ninety-Fourth Congress. First Session. U.S. Government Printing Office. Washington, D.C. January, 1975.

Recession and the Older Worker, The. Hearing Before the Subcommittee on Employment and Retirement Incomes. Special Committee on Aging. United States Senate. Ninety-Fourth Congress. First Session. Superintendent of Documents. U.S. Government Printing Office. Washington, D.C. 1976.

Resources After Retirement. U.S. Department of Health, Education, and Welfare. Social Security Administration. Office of Research and Statistics. Research Report No. 34. Superintendent of Documents. U.S. Government Printing Office. Washington, D.C. 1970.

Resources of People 65 or Over. Superintendent of Documents. U.S. Government Printing Office. Washington, D.C. 1971.

Schulz, James H. The Economic Status of the Retired Aged in 1980: Simulation Projections. Research Report No. 24. Superintendent of Documents. U.S. Government Printing Office. Washington, D.C. 1968.

Supplemental Security Program for the Aged, Blind and Disabled, The. U.S. Department of Health, Education, and Welfare. Social Security Administration. Office of Research and Statistics. Staff Paper, No. 17. Superintendent of Documents. U.S. Government Printing Office. Washington, D.C.

Tax Benefits for Older Americans, 1976. (Revised, October, 1975). Internal Revenue Service. U. S. Treasury Department. Publication No. 554. Superintendent of Documents. U. S. Government Printing Office. Washington, D. C.

Three Budgets For a Retired Couple in Urban Areas of the U.S., 1969-70. Bureau of Labor Statistics. Superintendent of Documents. U.S. Government Printing Office. Washington, D.C. 1971.

Wentworth, Edna C. and Motley, Dena K. _Resources After Retirement: A Study of Income, Assets and Living Arrangements of Social Security Beneficiaries, 1941 through 1962_. Social Security Administration. Office of Research and Statistics. Research Report No. 34. Superintendent of Documents. U.S. Government Printing Office. Washington, D.C. 1970.

Alford, Harold J. Continuing Education in Action: Residential Centers for Lifelong Learning. John Wiley and Sons, Inc. New York, New York. 1968.

A discussion of continuing education centers in large universities where the financial assistance is supported by the Kellogg Foundation.

Belbin, Eunice and Belbin, Meredith R. Problems in Adult Re-Training. National Council on the Aging. Washington, D.C. 1972.

A look at problems involved in retraining and discussion of responses by middle-aged recruits when exposed to different methods of training; suggestions are offered to those responsible for training programs.

Chandler, Suzannah. Home Maintenance and Repair Program For the Older Poor: A Model Community Action Program. National Council on the Aging. New York, New York. 1968.

A manual to aid in training the aged for repair and maintenance work in private homes of the elderly needing such service.

Consumer Education/Community College Bibliography. National Multimedia Center for Adult Education. Montclair State College. Upper Montclair, New Jersey. 1975.

A bibliography containing 160 abstracts on consumer education.

Consumer Handbook for Senior Citizens. Bureau of Business Research, College of Business and Economics, West Virginia University. Morgantown, West Virginia. 1975.

A practical guide, printed in large type for the older person. Information is included on services for the elderly, how to write letters of complaint, fraud, saving energy, credit, money management and Medicare.

Corbin, Dan H. and Tait, William J. Education for Leisure. Prentice-Hall, Inc. Englewood Cliffs, New Jersey. 1973.

Introduction to the field of leisure education and services with applicability for both the layman and the professional.

DeCrow, Roger. New Learning for Older Americans: An Overview of National Effort. Adult Education Association of the United States. Washington, D.C. 1975.

A summary of findings from questionnaires returned by 3500 agencies reporting learning opportunities for older adults. Aside from some special interests, the findings show the learning needs of old people are diverse and similar to needs of the rest of the population.

Entine, Alan (Editor). Americans in Middle Years: Career Options and Educational Opportunities. The Ethel Percy Andrus Gerontology Center. University of Southern California. Los Angeles, California. 1975.

A report of the views of twelve panelists at a conference held at State University of New York. The emphasis is on the challenges and opportunities of middle years.

Geba, Bruno. Vitality Training for Older Adults. Random House. New York, New York. 1974.

Dr. Geba advocates that the aged develop positive attitudes toward aging and challenges them to seek the necessary resources within themselves.

Gerontology Center: Education and Training in Aging; A Practical Guide for Professionals. Proceedings for First Report of the Region VIII Symposium for Trainers in Aging. Rocky Mountain Gerontology Center. Salt Lake City, Utah. 1975.

Title self explanatory.

Gobetz, Giles Edward, et al. Home Teaching of the Geriatric Blind. Cleveland Society for the Blind. Cleveland, Ohio. 1969.

Description and evaluation of a three-year study of home teaching project with the geriatric blind.

Grabowski, Stanley M. and Mason, W. Dean (Editors). *Education for the Aging*. Education Resources Division, Capitol Publications, Inc. Washington, D.C. (n.d.)

An anthology of recent literature and current practices in the field of education for the aging. Includes needs, practices, resources, extent of the field, and trends.

____. *Learning for Aging*. Adult Education Association of the U.S.A. Washington, D.C. 1974.

An analysis of learning, education and training among older persons; includes educational institution programs, innovative learning approaches, reports of research on learning among older Americans, and social implications.

Haak, Leo A. *A Comparative Analysis of the Institute Programs of the Oliver Wendell Holmes Association, 1963-1968*. New York, New York. 1969.

Description of adult education programs offered by the Association as coordinated effort in the communities or colleges. Students are retired and older persons.

Hendrickson, Andrew (Editor). *A Manual on Planning Educational Programs for Older Adults*. Department of Adult Education. Florida State University. Tallahassee, Florida. 1973.

A compilation of addresses from three Institutes on Education for Aging at Florida State University, 1969-1972, together with other materials. Topics cover the areas of understanding needs, counseling and teaching, planning and use of resources.

Heyman, Dorothy. *Community and Junior Colleges: Education and Training for Work with the Elderly*. Center for the Study of Aging and Human Development. Duke University Medical Center. Durham, N.C. 1975.

Proceedings of a conference on current program and community and junior college potential for meeting service needs of the elderly.

Hunter, Woodrow W. Preretirement Education for Hourly-rated Employees. University of Michigan. Division of Gerontology. Ann Arbor, Michigan. 1968.

A study designed to develop and test preretirement education material and methods for hourly paid workers, and to determine the effect of participation in a preretirement education program on both workers and their wives.

____________________. Preparation For Retirement. Revised edition. Institute of Gerontology. University of Michigan. Ann Arbor, Michigan. 1973.

Part one of this book discusses financial planning, health, and legal aspects of retirement; part two consists of short stories about typical retirement experiences.

Jacques, Joseph W. (Editor), Education for Aging Bibliography. Adult Continuing Education Center. Montclair State College. Upper Montclair, New Jersey. 1975.

A selected bibliography of abstracts from the National Multi-media Center for Adult Education.

Korim, Andrew S., et al. Older Americans and Community Colleges: A Guide for Program Implementation. American Association of Community and Junior Colleges. Washington, D.C. 1974.

A guide to community college involvement in public service in the field of aging and the relatively limited programming in this area.

Langerman, Philip D. (Editor), You Can Be Successful Teacher of Adults. National Association for Public Continuing and Adult Education. National Education Association. Washington, D.C. 1974.

An NAPCAE sourcebook and information guide for adult education and adult education teachers.

Lumsden, D. Barry and Sherron, Ronald H. (Editors). Experimental Studies in Adult Learning and Memory. Hemisphere Publishing Corporation. Washington, D.C. 1975.

A report on research and investigative studies dealing with adult learning and effects of aging on mental abilities, age related differentials, and other topics.

McGowan, Martin and McRoberts, Betty. *Seminars for Seniors: An Experiment in Educational Television for the Elderly*. Twin City Area Educational Television Corporation. St. Paul, Minnesota. (N.D.)

Analysis of an educational television series of programs for the elderly.

Never Too Old To Learn: A Report Submitted to the Edna McConnell Clark Foundation. Academy for Educational Development, Inc. New York, New York. 1974.

A study of available opportunities offered by post secondary institutions, reveals that few colleges and universities provide education and related services needed by the elderly. An annotated bibliography is included in this volume.

Older Americans and Community Colleges: An Overview. American Association of Community and Junior Colleges. Washington, D.C. 1974.

A brief report on the variety of ways in which community colleges are seeking to meet the needs of older persons in the communities they serve. Includes directory of community colleges and pertinent programs offered.

Rotrok, Lawrence and Miller, Linda DeAtley. *Active and Alert: Learning Experiences for Older Adults*. Missouri State Office on Aging. Jefferson City, Missouri. 1975.

A discussion of the adult learner and how he differs from younger students, and the implications for teaching methodology.

Vermilye, Dyckman W. (Editor). *Lifelong Learners: A New Clientele for Higher Education*. Jossey-Bass. San Francisco, California. 1974.

A report on the 29th National Conference on Higher Education held in Chicago, which treats changing trends in demands upon higher education resources and the lifelong needs and desires for educational opportunities.

U.S. GOVERNMENT PUBLICATIONS

An Approach to Consumer Education for Adults. Office of Consumer Affairs, Executive Office of the President. Washington, D.C. 1973.

Community Colleges Respond to Elders: Innovative Approaches Used. Bureau of Indian Affairs Schools. Office of Education. U. S. Department of Health, Education and Welfare. Superintendent of Documents. U. S. Government Printing Office. Washington, D. C. 1973.

Educationally Deficient Adults: Their Education and Training Needs. U.S. Office of Education. Superintendent of Documents. U.S. Government Printing Office. Washington, D.C. 1965.

Leiter, S. F. Training and Employment of the Older Worker. U.S. Department of Labor, Manpower Administration. Superintendent of Documents. U.S. Government Printing Office. Washington, D.C. 1968.

Lewis, Dorothea J. and Winsor, Richard J. Handle Yourself With Care. U.S. Department of Health, Education, and Welfare. Administration on Aging. Publication No. 804-IG. Superintendent of Documents. U.S. Government Printing Office. Washington, D.C. May, 1969.

Project Moneywise - Senior: Consumer Education for Older People. U.S. Department of Health, Education, and Welfare. Social and Rehabilitation Service. Administration on Aging. Washington, D.C. April, 1968.

EMPLOYMENT

Adams, Leonard P., et al. Employment of the Middle-Aged Worker. National Council on the Aging. Washington, D.C. 1969.

Investigation of some new and pressing questions faced by older people in the American work force including, employment opportunities, adaptability to new types of jobs, involuntary early retirement, and the effects of technology on older workers.

Albee, Lou. Over Forty---Out of Work? How to Win at the Job Hunting Game. Prentice-Hall. Englewood Cliffs, New Jersey. 1970.

Facts and suggestions pertaining to the problems of the unemployed older person.

Angel, Juvenal L. Employment Opportunities for Men and Women After 60. Regents Publishing Co. New York, New York. 1969.

General discussion of older workers, their career opportunities, and special occupational problems.

Clague, Ewan, et al. The Aging Worker and the Union: Employment and Retirement of Middle-Aged and Older Workers. Praeger Publishers, Inc. New York, New York. 1971.

A survey of the policies and practices of organized labor with respect to older workers in unions. The main objective of this inquiry was to discover the variety of ways in which unions have approached the interests of older workers.

Clark, Frederick LeGros. Work, Age and Leisure. Michael Joseph Publishers. London, England. 1966.

Discussion of the causes and consequences of the shortened working life.

Dirken, J. M. (Editor). Functional Age of Industrial Workers. International Scholarly Book Services. Portland, Oregon. 1972.

A report of a multidisciplinary research project on working capacity and aging. The findings of this study provide objective criteria for the formulation of personnel policy in respect to retirement on a basis other than calendar age.

Elderly Services and Industries: An Evaluation of a Program of Paid, Part-time Employment for Elderly Poor. Center for Urban Studies. University of Akron. Akron, Ohio. 1970.

Report on a three year pilot project conducted by the government at Martin's Ferry, Ohio, where 28 elderly persons were employed in five work programs.

Guidelines for the Development of Employment Opportunities for Older People. National Council on the Aging. Washington, D.C. 1971.

Description of the Senior Community Service Project, with findings demonstrating the employability of older persons in a non-professional capacity in community service agencies.

Heidbreder, Elizabeth M. Middle-Aged and Older Workers in Industry. (Facts and Trends No. 1) National Council on the Aging. 1973.

Statements pertaining to the hiring, training, retraining, retirement policies, and pensions of the middle-aged and older worker.

Impact of Technological Change on Older Workers in the International Typographical Union: A Case Study. National Council on the Aging. Washington, D.C. 1973.

Monograph reporting on the change from linotype printing to cold print, and how older workers learned new methods and assumed new job roles.

Industrial Gerontology: An Annotated Bibliography on Industrial Change and Aging in the Work Force. National Institute of Industrial Gerontology. National Council on Aging. Washington, D. C. 1968.

References include research findings on aging in the work force, private pension plans, employment data by age groups, discrimination, older worker potentials, and other topics.

Jaffe, A. J. The Middle Years, Neither Too Young Nor Too Old. National Council on the Aging. Washington, D.C. 1972.

A discussion of Americans in their middle years; including work, educational backgrounds, family structure and ability to make a living, income changes, and health.

Kelleher, Carol H. Second Careers. National Council on the Aging. Washington, D.C. 1973.

Ideas for mid-life and retirement career changes.

Koyl, Leon F. Employing the Older Worker: Matching the Employee to the Job. Second Edition. National Council on the Aging. Washington, D.C. 1974.

Analysis and explanation of the Gulhemp system for objectively measuring worker abilities to fulfill job requirements, a tool for matching the worker to the job and the job to the worker.

____________ and Hanson, Pamela Marsters. Age, Physical Ability, and Work Potential. National Council on the Aging. Washington, D.C. 1969.

A description of two measurement techniques designed to determine the physical and emotional fitness of a worker for a specific job.

Kreps, Juanita M. (Editor). Employment, Income, and Retirement Problems of the Aged. Duke University. Durham, North Carolina. 1968.

Trends in income, employment, and labor force size, and the relations of these trends to changing age structure of the population. First printed in 1963.

____________ (Editor). Technology, Manpower, and Retirement Policy. World Publishing Company. Cleveland, Ohio. 1966.

A discussion of problems confronting workers which arise from policies designed to reduce the size of the labor force.

____________ and Clark, Robert. Sex, Age and Work. John Hopkins University Press. Baltimore, Maryland. 1976.

The purpose of this book has been to give attention to the changing composition of the labor force and of the reallocation of time devoted to "market work, home work and leisure." Conclusions consider the effects upon manpower policies.

Lewis, Adele, and Bobroff, Edith. From Kitchen to Career. The Bobbs-Merrill Publishing Company. Indianapolis, Indiana. 1968.

Job hunting advice for older women.

Liebers, Arthur. How to Start A Profitable Retirement Business. Pilot Books. New York, New York. 1968.

Ideas for small investment businesses, many of which can be operated part time and from the home.

Luchterhand, Elmer, and Sydiaha, Daniel. Choice in Human Affairs: An Application to Aging - Accident - Illness Problems. College and University Press. New Haven, Connecticut. 1966.

Description of a project relocating blue collar workers in jobs following partial loss of physical capacity due to aging, accidents or illness.

National Seminar on Aging: Served by and Serving as Sub-professionals, Proceedings. American Public Welfare Association. Chicago, Illinois. 1970.

Discussion of ways and means for using old people to deliver services to the aged.

Rusalem, Herbert. The Vocational Adjustment of the Older Disabled Worker: A Selective Review of Recent Literature. Federation Employment and Guidance Service. New York, New York. 1966.

A mongraph delineating major factors conditioning employment of older disabled and non-disabled workers. Includes an extensive list of references.

Second Careers. National Council on the Aging. Washington, D. C. Revised periodically.

An annotated bibliography.

Shatto, Gloria M. (Editor). Employment of the Middle-Aged: Papers from Industrial Gerontology Seminars. Charles C. Thomas. Springfield, Illinois. 1972.

A collection of papers analyzing various aspects of employment problems and opportunities facing middle-aged and older persons. The writers explore attitudes and financial provisions, elaborate on policy objectives, and suggest legislation changes related to employment and the aged.

Sheppard, Harold L. New Perspectives on Older Workers, The. W. E. Upjohn Institute for Employment Research. Kalamazoo, Michigan. 1971.

Collection of papers on industrial gerontology, including report of studies on problems of older workers, socioeconomic factors related to status of white women and urban blacks, second careers; suggests role of behavioral science in problem solving.

________________ (Editor). Towards an Industrial Gerontology: An Introduction to A New Field of Applied Research and Service. Schenkman Publishing Company. Cambridge, Massachusetts. 1970.

A series of papers presented at the 1968 Seminar on Industrial Gerontology which included aptitude testing of middle aged and older workers, employment counseling, retirement adjustment, and public and private pensions.

Small, Samuel. Starting A Business After 50. Pilot Books. New York, New York. 1974.

Guidelines for the older person wanting to start a new business.

Spear, Mel. The Guide for In-Service Training for Older Persons: A Report of the APWA-California Project. American Public Welfare Association. Public Welfare Project on Aging. Chicago, Illinois. 1970.

A monograph which reports experiences in a project with the elderly; includes concepts related to the aging process.

Sprague, N. (Editor). Industrial Gerontology. No. 2. National Council on the Aging. Washington, D. C. June, 1969.

This volume includes an emphasis upon the range of factors that affect older workers.

Welford, A. T., and Birren, J. E. Interdisciplinary Topics in Gerontology: VI: Decision Making and Age. NATO Advanced Study Institute. University of Thessalonika, 1967. S. Karger Publishers. New York, New York. 1969.

An international perspective on aging with a particular emphasis upon work performance, work choice and psychological aspects.

"Working In Retirement." The Retirement Living Magazine. 150 East 58th Street, New York, New York 10022. 1975.

This publication, equivalent to a monograph, reports a study on why people continue to work after retirement, how they find employment, types of employment. Drawing upon these data, there are guidelines for planning, resources available and work status of the older worker.

U. S. GOVERNMENT PUBLICATIONS

Age Discrimination in Employment Act of 1967, As Amended. Wage and Hour Division. Labor Department. Superintendent of Documents. U. S. Government Printing Office. Washington, D. C. 1975.

Back to Work After Retirement. U. S. Department of Labor. Manpower Administration. Superintendent of Documents. U. S. Government Printing Office. Washington, D. C. 1972.

Carrera, Anna F. Age Discrimination in Employment Act of 1967. Employment Standards Administration. U. S. Department of Labor. Washington, D. C. 1974.

Employment Aspects of the Economics of Aging: A Working Paper in Conjunction With the Overall Study of Economics of Aging; Toward A Full Share in Abundance. National Institute of Industrial Gerontology. Ninety-first Congress. First Session. Superintendent of Documents. U. S. Government Printing Office. Washington, D. C. 1969.

Fair Labor Standards Amendments of 1974 (P.L. 93-259) Showing Changes Made in Fair Labor Standards Act of 1938, As Amended; Portal to Portal Pay Act of 1947; and Age Discrimination in Employment Act of 1967. Subcommittee on Labor. Labor and Public Welfare Committee. Ninety-third Congress. Second Session. U. S. Senate. Washington, D. C. 1974.

Flexitime: A Handbook for Managers and Employees Who Want to Know More About Developing A Flexible Work Schedule. U. S. Civil Service Commission. Superintendent of Documents. U. S. Government Printing Office. Washington, D. C. 1974.

Heidbreder, Elizabeth. Cancelled Careers: The Impact of Reduction-In-Force Policies on Middle-Aged Federal Employees. A Report to the Special Committee on Aging. U. S. Congress. United States Senate. Superintendent of Documents. U. S. Government Printing Office. Washington, D. C. 1972.

Improving Age Discrimination Law: Working Paper. Special Committee on Aging. Ninety-third Congress. First Session. United States Senate. Superintendent of Documents. U. S. Government Printing Office. Washington, D. C. 1973.

Job Redesign for Older Workers: Ten Case Studies. U. S. Bureau of Labor Statistics. Superintendent of Documents. U. S. Government Printing Office. Washington, D. C. 1967.

Leiter, Sarah F. Training and Employment of the Older Worker: Recent Findings and Recommendations Based on Older Worker Experimental and Demonstration Projects. U. S. Manpower Administration. Washington, D. C. 1968.

Nation's Stake in the Employment of Middle-Aged and Older Persons, The. Special Committee on Aging. United States Senate. Superintendent of Documents. U. S. Government Printing Office. Washington, D. C. July, 1971.

Older Americans Community Service Employment Act. Committee on Labor and Public Welfare. Ninety-second Congress. U. S. Senate. Superintendent of Documents. U. S. Government Printing Office. Washington, D. C. 1972.

Parnes, Herbert S., et al (Editors). Pre-Retirement Years, The. Report of Longitudinal Study of the Labor Market Experience of Men. U. S. Department of Labor. Manpower Research Monograph No. 15. U. S. Government Printing Office. Washington, D. C.

Vol. 1 - 1970
Vol. 2 - 1970
Vol. 3 - 1973

Perales, Gabriel, Jr. Age Discrimination in Employment Act of 1967. Employment Standards Administration. U. S. Labor Department. Superintendent of Documents. U. S. Government Printing Office. Washington, D. C. 1972.

Recommended for Action: Employment and Retirement. White House Conference on Aging. Superintendent of Documents. U. S. Government Printing Office. Washington, D. C. 1972.

Unemployment Among Older Workers. Subcommittee on Employment and Retirement Incomes. Special Committee on Aging. Ninety-second Congress. First Session. United States Senate. Superintendent of Documents. U. S. Government Printing Office. Washington, D. C. 1972.

Wentworth, Edna C. Employment After Retirement: A Study of the Post-entitlement Work Experience of Men Drawing Benefits Under Social Security. Research Report No. 21. Superintendent of Documents. U. S. Government Printing Office. Washington, D. C. 1968.

ETHNIC GROUPS

Balkema, John B. The Aged in Minority Groups: A Bibliography. The National Council on the Aging, Inc. Washington, D. C. 1973.

An annotated bibliography dealing with the relatively small body of literature on minority group aged.

Battle, Mark (Editor). Employment Prospects of Aged Blacks, Chicanos and Indians. National Council on the Aging. Washington, D. C. 1971.

Description of experiences of people who are elderly, poor, and also members of an ethnic minority group.

Brennan, Jere L. The Forgotten American -- American Indians Remembered: A Selected Bibliography for Use in Social Work Education. Council on Social Work Education. New York, New York. 1972.

An annotated bibliography prepared as a resource for better understanding the American Indian.

Cohen, Elias, et al. Minority Aged in America. Occasional Papers in Gerontology. Institute of Gerontology. University of Michigan. Ann Arbor, Michigan. 1973.

An analysis of the plight of America's aged black and Indian populations.

Coles, Robert. The Old Ones of New Mexico. University of New Mexico Press. Albuquerque, New Mexico. Doubleday Anchor Press. New York, New York. 1973.

A perceptive treatment by text and photographs of one group of older Americans.

Davis, Richard H. (Editor). Health Services and the Mexican-American Elderly. Ethel Percy Andrus Gerontology Center. University of Southern California Press. Los Angeles, California. 1973.

A monograph of conference transcriptions. Participants included citizens, panelists, and health care professionals.

Davis, Richard M. (Editor). *Community Services and the Black Elderly*. Andrus Gerontology Center. University of Southern California. Los Angeles, California. 1972.

A collection of papers prepared for training service workers with elderly black persons. Offers brief coverage of a number of topics, including use of time, health services, social services.

Jewish Community Plan for the Elderly, A. Gerontological Council, Jewish Federation of Metropolitan Chicago. The Federation. Chicago, Illinois. 1970.

A report on the needs of aged residents of Chicago and services provided to Jewish aged. Includes recommendations for better coordinated, comprehensive service programs for elderly Jews.

Kent, Donald P. *Social, Economic and Health Conditions of Negroes and White Aged and Their Utilization of Community Resources*. Pennsylvania State University. University Park, Pennsylvania. 1970.

A monograph reporting existing conditions together with documentary case histories, statistical reports and other relevant information.

Kiefer, Christie. *Changing Cultures, Changing Lives*. Jossey-Bass, Inc. San Francisco, California. 1974.

An analysis of the cultural conflict among Japanese-Americans based upon observation and interviews with immigrants, their children, and their grandchildren.

Moore, Joan W. *Mexican Americans*. Prentice-Hall, Inc. Englewood Cliffs, New Jersey. 1970. (Ethnic Groups in American Life Series)

A documentary report on one of the largest minority groups in the United States, about whom relatively little is known.

Rabinowitz, Dorothy. *The Other Jews: Portraits in Poverty*. The American Jewish Committee. Institute of Human Relations Press. New York, New York. 1972.

A monograph depicting eight elderly Jewish poor who are isolated and sick. Action needed is evident.

Reich, J. M., et al. Relocating the Dispossessed Elderly: A Study of Mexican Americans. Institute for Environmental Studies. University of Pennsylvania. Philadelphia, Pennsylvania. 1966.

Study of inadequate community planning and lack of understanding of needs of elderly Mexican Americans relocated in San Antonio, Texas.

Stanford, E. Percil (Editor). Minority Aging: Proceedings. Center on Aging. San Diego State University. San Diego, California. 1974.

The proceedings of an Institute on Minority Aging held in 1973. Treats the problems and circumstances of the old among minority groups and quality of their lives.

Steglich, W. G., et al. Survey of Needs and Resources Among Aged Mexican Americans: Final Report. Texas Governor's Committee on Aging. Texas Technological College. Lubbock, Texas. 1968.

Report on a survey to determine attitudes toward old age by older Mexican Americans, and attitudes toward support from the family, the church and the government.

Triple Jeopardy: Myth or Reality. National Council on the Aging. Washington, D. C. 1972.

Four papers from NCOA regional meetings on problems of aged American Indians, blacks, rural whites and Spanish speaking people.

Weeks, H. Ashley, and Darsky, Benjamin J. The Urban Aged: Race and Medical Care. School of Public Health. Bureau of Public Health. Economics Research Series No. 14. University of Michigan. Ann Arbor, Michigan. 1968.

Study of the differential use of health services by subgroups of aged, with particular attention to the urban Negro aged. The differences in need and use of out-of-pocket expenditures for medical care are explored.

U. S. GOVERNMENT PUBLICATIONS

Advisory Council on the Elderly American Indian: A Statement by Council Members, Together With Analyses of Available Statistical Information and Other Appendix Material. Special Committee on Aging. United States Senate. Superintendent of Documents. U. S. Government Printing Office. Washington, D. C. 1971.

Availibility and Usefulness of Federal Programs and Services to Elderly Mexican Americans. Special Committee on Aging. United States Senate. Superintendent of Documents. U. S. Government Printing Office. Washington, D. C. 1969-1970. (5 Volumes).

Kaplan, Hirsch, and Taylor, Benjamin J. Economic and Social Problems of the Elderly Urban Indian in Phoenix, Arizona. Administration on Aging. U. S. Department of Health, Education and Welfare. Washington, D. C. 1972.

Multiple Hazards of Age and Race: The Situation of Aged Blacks in the United States, The. A Preliminary Survey for the Special Committee on Aging. United States Senate. Ninety-Second Congress. First Session. Superintendent of Documents. U. S. Government Printing Office. Washington, D. C. September, 1971.

Recommended for Action: Aging and Aged Blacks. White House Conference on Aging. Superintendent of Documents. U. S. Government Printing Office. Washington, D. C. 1972.

Recommended For Action: Asian American Elderly. White House Conference on Aging. Superintendent of Documents. U. S. Government Printing Office. Washington, D. C. 1972.

Recommended for Action: Elderly Indian. White House Conference on Aging. Superintendent of Documents. U. S. Government Printing Office. Washington, D. C. 1972.

Reyes, Manolo. Elderly Cubans in Exile. Special Committee on Aging. Ninety-Second Congress. First Session. United States Senate. Superintendent of Documents. U. S. Government Printing Office. Washington, D. C. 1971.

Reynoso, Cruz, and Coppelman, Peter D. Proposals to Eliminate Legal Barriers Affecting Elderly Mexican-Americans. Special Committee on Aging. Ninety-Second Congress. Second Session. United States Senate. Superintendent of Documents. U. S. Government Printing Office. Washington, D. C. 1972.

Spanish Speaking Elderly. White House Conference on Aging. Superintendent of Documents. U. S. Government Printing Office. Washington, D. C. 1971.

FAMILY AND FAMILY RELATIONS

Bengtson, Vern L. (Editor). Intergenerational Relations. Ethel Percy Andrus Gerontology Center. University of Southern California. Los Angeles, California.

A bibliography.

Beresford, John C., et al. Living in the Multigeneration Family. Occasional Papers in Gerontology, No. 3. Institute of Gerontology. University of Michigan-Wayne State University. Ann Arbor, Michigan. 1969.

Essays on the four-generation family, including demographic data, financial considerations, interpersonal relations, crisis of widowhood, and the grandparent role.

Coakley, Mary Lewis. When Parents Grow Old. Franciscan Publishers. Pulaski, Wisconsin. 1967.

Consideration of living arrangements and mental and physical conditions of aging parents. Constructive actions are suggested.

Family Is All Generations, The. Family Service Association of America. New York, New York. 1965.

Suggestions of ways to assist old people and their families in multigeneration living.

Field, Minna. The Aged, the Family, and the Community. Columbia University Press. New York, New York. 1972.

Discussion of impact of unfavorable economic, social, and health conditions on self image and relationships with family. Suggestions are offered for positive change.

Fritz, Dorothy Bertolet. Growing Old Is A Family Affair. John Knox Press. Richmond, Virginia. 1972.

The audience for this book is primarily persons in their middle years since they are chiefly responsible for training the young and providing care for the aged.

Koller, Marvin R. Families: A Multigenerational Approach. McGraw-Hill Book Company. New York, New York. 1974.

In addition to such topics as interpersonal relations, generational responsibilities, and similar topics usually considered under this title, family life in middle and old age is discussed. Also an analysis of the effect of family heritage on present and future generations.

McKain, Walter C. Retirement and Marriage. Storrs Agricultural Experiment Station. University of Connecticut. Storrs, Connecticut. 1969.

A comprehensive and insightful study of 100 recently married elderly couples; explores the courtship, marriage ceremony, reasons for marriage, and factors related to their success.

Older Person In the Family: Challenges and Conflict. Proceedings of Conference on Gerontology. Institute of Gerontology. University of Iowa. Iowa City, Iowa. 1965.

A realistic consideration of the role of the older person in a family unit.

Otten, Jane, and Shelley, Florence D. When Your Parents Grow Old. Funk and Wagnalls. Binghamton, New York. 1977.

This book was written for adult children as a resource in dealing with problems of their aged parents. Provides guidance and information.

Peterson, James Alfred. Married Love In the Middle Years. Association Press. New York, New York. 1968.

Consideration of the many aspects of adjustment associated with middle age.

Poe, William D. The Old Person in Your Home. Charles Scribner's Sons. New York, New York. 1969.

A physician writes for lay audience, incorporating practical information on a variety of the components of care and daily living.

Richardson, Frank Howard. Grandparents and Their Families: A Guide for Three Generations. McKay. New York, New York. 1964.

Ways to promote a happier relationship among grandparents, parents, and grandchildren.

Shanas, Ethel, and Streib, Gordon F. (Editors). Social Structure and the Family: Generational Relations. Prentice-Hall, Inc. Englewood Cliffs, New Jersey. 1965.

A cross-cultural perspective of the three-generation family structure in Western society, with particular emphasis on generational relationships of old family members. It coordinates views from the fields of psychiatry, economics, and sociology.

Stern, Edith M., and Ross, Mabel. You and Your Aging Parents. Harper and Row Publishers, Inc. New York, New York. 1965.

A practical guide for those who have a sincere interest in their parents, while also fulfilling responsibilities to themselves and their families.

Townsend, Peter. The Family Life of Old People. Penguin Books. Baltimore, Maryland. 1963.

Study of old people in Bethnal Green, a suburb of East London. First reported in 1957. Although old, this work still contains many useful insights.

GERIATRIC MEDICINE

Altamura, Michael V., et al. Aging Patients, A Guide for Their Care. Springer Publishing Company. New York, New York. 1976.

The authors, a physician and two registered nurses, have written a handbook for paraprofessionals which includes: aging changes, disease entities and their treatment, medical terminology, and various physical therapies and their use.

Anderson, W. F., and Judge, T. G. (Editors). Geriatric Medicine. Academic Press. New York, New York. 1974.

Directed primarily to persons engaged in clinical research, this volume covers not only medical topics, but also psychology, education and sociology; could be helpful to medical students who gain little exposure to geriatric medicine in their formal training.

Bab, Werner. The Uses of Psychology in Geriatric Ophthalmology. Charles C. Thomas. Springfield, Illinois. 1964.

A short guide for the ophthalmologist, general practitioner, and others who see and treat elderly people in professional practice.

Berezin, Martin, A., and Cath, Stanley H. (Editors). Geriatric Psychiatry: Grief, Loss, and Emotional Disorders in the Aging Process. International Universities Press, Inc. New York, New York. 1967.

Title self explanatory.

Brocklehurst, John C. (Editor). Geriatric Care in Advanced Societies. University Park Press. Baltimore, Maryland. 1975.

A review by qualified authorities of how geriatric care problems are being solved in the United States, England, Australia, Europe and the Soviet Union; emphasis is upon medical problems associated with increased longevity.

__________________. Textbook of Geriatric Medicine and Gerontology. Longman, Inc. New York, New York. 1973.

An authoritative textbook in which 44 authors give information on geriatric medicine and gerontology. The publication is divided into three sections: biological gerontology, clinical geriatric medicine, and socio-psychological gerontology. Includes also a discussion of medical care for the elderly.

Busse, Ewald W. (Editor). _Theory and Therapeutics of Aging_. Medcom Press. New York, New York. 1973.

A book which attempts to provide some perspective on the aging process related to medicine; discusses skills currently available and future expectations. A valuable volume to researchers and practicing physicians concerned with the aging process.

______________ , and Pfeiffer, Eric (Editors). _Mental Illness in Later Life_. American Psychiatric Association. Washington, D. C. 1973.

A brief, clear delineation of information practicing physicians need in order to diagnose and treat aged patients. Part one deals with the social, psychological and economic environment as well as prevention, diagnosis and treatment of disability. Part two is a compilation of questions and answers about problems of aging frequently asked by health professionals.

Coons, Dorothy H. _The Process of Change_. Institute of Gerontology. University of Michigan. Ann Arbor, Michigan. 1973.

A discussion of the administrator's role in the orderly transformation of an institutional environment into one that promotes a treatment program for older persons.

Cowdry, E. V., and Steinberg, Franz U. (Editors). _The Care of the Geriatric Patient_. Fifth Edition. The C. V. Mosby Company. St. Louis, Missouri. 1976.

A summary of the wide variety of information essential to those who care for the geriatric patient.

Ehrlich, George Edward. _Total Management of the Arthritic Patient_. J. B. Lippincott Company. Philadelphia, Pennsylvania. 1973.

A comprehensive treatment of therapy needs of arthritic patients, with the primary attention given to rheumatoid arthritis.

Elliott, Neil. _The Gods of Life_. Macmillan Publishing Company, Inc. New York, New York. 1974.

A comparison of treatment of the aged in the past with treatment by modern societies. Discusses problems associated with new technologies, e.g., medical prolongation of life, hospital and nursing home quality of care, euthanasia controversies, and the public health system as it relates to extent of care for the aged.

Felstein, Ivor. Later Life: Geriatrics Today and Tomorrow. Penguin Books. Baltimore, Maryland. 1969.

Emphasis is upon need for the specialty of geriatrics in medicine, and the fact that the need will not diminish. Included are ideas on care of the elderly, various types of hospitals and health delivery models and preventive geriatric care.

______________. Living to be A Hundred: A Study of Old Age. Hippocrene Books, Inc. New York, New York. 1973.

A non-technical discussion of modern geriatric medical care.

Freeman, Joseph T. (Editor). Clinical Features of the Older Patient. Charles C. Thomas. Springfield, Illinois. 1965.

A presentation of the interrelated mechanisms, morphological, and physiological, and their adaptive nature to senescent demands.

Gaitz, Charles M., et al. Goals of Comprehensive Health Care in Advanced Old Age. Institute of Gerontology. University of Michigan-Wayne State University. Ann Arbor, Michigan. 1968.

Monograph dealing with medical and psychological health care of the elderly and goals established to provide more comprehensive clinical management of older persons.

Galton, Lawrence. Don't Give Up On An Aging Parent. Crown Publishers. New York, New York. 1975.

Discussion of commonly held myths about diseases among old people and an examination of modern medical care and care needs of the aged.

Geist, Harold. The Psychological Aspects of Rheumatoid Arthritis. Charles C. Thomas. Springfield, Illinois. 1966.

The etiology and treatment of rheumatoid arthritis from a psychological perspective.

Gershon, Samuel, and Raskin, Allen (Editors). Genesis and Treatment of Psychologic Disorders in the Elderly. (Vol. 2 of Series on Aging). Raven Press. New York, New York. 1975.

A compilation of research related to the development and treatment of psychologic disorders in older persons. It provides a reference in the new field of geriatric psychobiology, combining a report of basic studies and clinical investigations.

Greenfield, Lazar J. *Surgery of the Aged*. Vol. 17 in the series, "Major Problems in Clinical Surgery." W. B. Saunders Company. Philadelphia, Pennsylvania. 1975.

A book for physicians dealing specifically with the special considerations required for older adults.

Harris, Raymond. *The Management of Geriatric Cardiovascular Disease*. J. B. Lippincott Company. Philadelphia, Pennsylvania. 1970.

Coverage includes management, as well as diagnosis, treatment and rehabilitation of the aged patient suffering from cardiovascular disease.

Hazell, Kenneth. *Social and Medical Problems of the Elderly*. Third Edition. Hutchinson Medical Publications. London, England. 1973.

Discussion of problems in care of the elderly; practical solutions for some problems associated with care of the aged, and emphasis on preventive medicine and hospital care.

Health Care for Older People. National Council on the Aging. Washington, D. C. Revised periodically.

An annotated bibliography.

Hodkinson, H. M. *An Outline of Geriatrics*. Academic Press. New York, New York. 1975.

A monograph directed to medical students which touches briefly upon a number of topics related to medical care of geriatric patients.

Homburger, Freddy, and Bonner, Charles D. *Medical Care and Rehabilitation of the Aged and Chronically Ill*. Third Edition. Little, Brown and Company. Boston, Massachusetts. 1974.

Two major topics are discussed: 1) therapeutic procedures for use with aged patients and those with selected chronic diseases, and 2) the roles of professionals and family in effective therapy.

Howell, Trevor. *Old Age. Some Practical Points in Geriatrics*. Third Edition. H. K. Lewis Publishers. London, England. 1974.

A short book on geriatrics which is divided into three parts: Clinical, Morbid Anatomy, and Administration.

Howell, Trevor H. A Student's Guide to Geriatrics. Charles C. Thomas. Springfield, Illinois. 1970.

Good introductory book on geriatric medicine which can be understood by the layman. Age related changes are discussed, and attention is given to community service organizations.

Howells, John G. (Editor). Modern Perspectives in the Psychiatry of Old Age. Brunner/Mazel, Inc. New York, New York. 1975.

A comprehensive cross-cultural summary of psychiatry as it applies to old age. Topics covered include genetics, epidemiology, neurosis, depression, suicide, functional psychosis, and other topics in the growing field of psychogeriatrics.

Hyams, Dennis. The Care of the Aged. Health Science Division. Technomic Publishing Company. Westport, Connecticut. 1976.

This book is comprised of a section on old age and geriatric problems with need for total patient care rather than fragmentation in care. A second section includes case histories and other medical considerations, e.g., death and dying, euthanasia.

Irvine, R. E., et al. The Older Geriatric Patient: An Introduction to Geriatrics. Second Edition. English Universities Press. London, England. 1970.

Geriatric care is discussed by a physician, a nurse, and a medical social worker.

Isaacs, B., et al. Survival of the Unfittest: A Study of Geriatric Patients in Glasgow. Routledge & Kegan Paul, Ltd. Boston, Massachusetts. 1972.

This book reports the findings of a survey comparing geriatric and other medical patients in respect to physical and mental incapacities as well as definitive disease entities.

Jaeger, Dorothea, and Simmons, Leo W. The Aged Ill: Coping With Problems in Geriatric Care. Appleton-Century-Crofts. New York, New York. 1970.

An identification of crucial problems in coping with illness and infirmity in old age and with the terminally ill; offers suggestions for meeting needs.

LaRue, Vivien. Two Years With Eighty Patients. Resources in Aging. Institute of Gerontology. University of Michigan. Ann Arbor, Michigan. 1973.

Report on attempts to transform a traditional mental hospital geriatric ward into one offering a treatment program.

Lawson, Ian R., and Ingman, Stanley R. (Editors). The Language of Geriatric Care: Implication for Professional Review. Connecticut Health Services Research Series. North Haven, Connecticut. 1975.

This report of the proceedings of a University of Connecticut School of Medicine Conference concentrates on developing a better clinical science for dealing with clinical problems of elderly persons. Topics include rehabilitation, problem oriented medical records, toxonomy of disease and geriatric care, among others.

Levitt, Eugene E., and Lubin, Bernard. Depression. Springer Publishing Company. New York, New York. 1975.

Report of a study based on a random survey of the general population, relating depression to age, race, sex, and socio-economic status. Depression is treated as a separate diagnostic entity.

Lidz, Theodore. The Person. Basic Books, Inc. New York, New York. 1968.

The sequence of growth and development from birth to death is related to behavior. In the chapter dealing specifically with old age, the author discusses the problem created by medical science with regard to the rapid growth of the older population and its social impact, and the concomitant disregard of the need for medical practice to adjust to the changing population needs.

Lilienfeld, Abraham M., and Gifford, Alice J. Chronic Diseases and Public Health. Johns Hopkins Press. Baltimore, Maryland. 1966.

Several chapters are included on care of long-term patients and the economic problems involved.

Lorhan, Paul H. Anesthesia for the Aged. Charles C. Thomas. Springfield, Illinois. 1971.

Effective presentation of problems encountered in use of anesthesia for aged patients.

Metzelaar, Lena. Social Interaction Groups In A Therapeutic Community. Resources in Aging. Institute of Gerontology. University of Michigan. Ann Arbor, Michigan. 1973.

A description of techniques which have proved effective in working with geriatric mental patients.

Miller, Michael B. The Interdisciplinary Role of the Nursing Home Medical Director. Contemporary Publishing, Inc. Wakefield, Massachusetts. 1975.

The author defines the parameters for medical programs for care of aged persons in long term care institutions. Included is the importance of interrelationships of professional roles in care.

"Physician's Role in the Care of the Aging, The." Symposium Proceedings. The Gerontologist, Vol. 10, No. 2. The Gerontological Society. Washington, D. C. 1970.

Title self explanatory.

Planning and Organization of Geriatric Services: Report of a WHO Expert Committee. World Health Organization Technical Report Series, No. 548. World Health Organization. Geneva, Switzerland. 1974.

A helpful guide for nations and organizations interested in providing services to the aged.

Powers, John H. (Editor). Surgery of the Aged and Debilitated Patient. W. B. Saunders Company. Philadelphia, Pennsylvania. 1968.

Topics covered are physiology of aging, the pathogenesis of diseases in old age, and the metabolic management of geriatric surgical patients.

Ramsey, Paul. The Patient As Person: Explorations in Medical Ethics. Yale University Press. New Haven, Connecticut. 1972.

An examination of some of the current problems of medical ethics such as, the ethics of consent, procedures for identifying death, and care of the dying, as well as the giving of vital organs and the giving or taking of cadaver organs for transplants.

Rappaport, Julian, et al. Innovations in Helping Chronic Patients. Academic Press. New York, New York. 1971.

Description of an experimental program in community mental health using college students as group leaders to help in the treatment of chronic mentally ill patients.

Rossman, Isadore (Editor). Clinical Geriatrics. J. B. Lippincott Company. Philadelphia, Pennsylvania. 1971.

Title self explanatory.

Rubin, Ira Lloyd, et al. Treatment of Heart Disease in the Adult. Second Edition. Lea and Febiger. Philadelphia, Pennsylvania. 1972.

A text written for clinicians; discusses types of heart disease and their treatment.

Seminar on Administrative Development: Licensure and Gerontology. Proceedings. Division of Economic and Business Research. College of Business and Public Administration. University of Arizona. Tucson, Arizona. 1970.

An overview of problems in medical care, nursing homes, and administration.

Sigel, Michael M., and Good, Robert A. Tolerance, Autoimmunity and Aging. Charles C. Thomas. Springfield, Illinois. 1972.

Physical aging topics include age related change, disease and spontaneous autoimmunity. Reports are made on animal research.

Simon, Alexander, et al. Crisis and Intervention. Jossey-Bass, Inc. San Francisco, California. 1970.

Descriptive analysis of 543 aged urban residents hospitalized during a single calendar year for extreme psychiatric disorders.

Solomons, Bethel. Skin Care. Health Science Division. Technomic Publishing Company. Westport, Connecticut. 1976.

The author, a dermatologist, writes on skin disorders and treatment at all ages, with a special attention to aging skin.

Sperber, Perry A. Treatment of the Aging Skin and Dermal Defects. Charles C. Thomas. Springfield, Illinois. 1965.

Title self explanatory.

Steinberg, Franz U. (Editor). Cowdry's the Care of the Geriatric Patient. Fifth Edition. The C. V. Mosby Company. St. Louis, Missouri. 1976.

Forty-three contributors advise on all aspects of medical and surgical care of aged patients, disorders commonly found, rehabilitation and psychological and social aspects of care.

Stewart, Monnica C. My Brother's Keeper? Second Edition. Health Horizon, Limited, for the Chest and Heart Association. London, England. 1971.

A discussion of the geriatric wards in British hospitals. Considers care of the aged from medical, psychological, societal, family and community viewpoints.

Stone, LaRue, and Lamb, Lawrence E. There's Help for Arthritis. Enterprise Publications. New York, New York. 1971.

Written by a physician with arthritis, the book offers practical help, information and encouragement to patients with rheumatoid arthritis.

Stotsky, Bernard Alexandrovich. The Elderly Patient. Grune and Stratton, Inc. New York, New York. 1968.

A summary of findings from psychiatric and behavioral science studies of the elderly patient. Some attention is given to service programs for the elderly.

________________________. The Nursing Home and the Aged Psychiatric Patient. Appleton-Century-Crofts. New York, New York. 1970.

A guide for therapeutic management of emotionally disturbed residents of nursing homes.

Strauss, Anselm L. Chronic Illness and the Quality of Life. The C. V. Mosby Company. St. Louis, Missouri. 1975.

The emphasis of this book is upon ill persons of all ages in the home, and the social-psychological aspects of living with a chronic disability. One section is devoted to a study of several specific chronic illnesses, with a final section related to the health care field and patient care.

Summit, Leon (Editor). The Crisis in Health Care for the Aging. The Huxley Institute for Biosocial Research. New York, New York. 1973.

Report of a national conference in 1972 designed to increase public awareness and understanding of the needs and of the possibilities for improvement in health care for the elderly.

Toward a Public Policy on Mental Health Care of the Elderly. Vol. VII, No. 79. Group for the Advancement of Psychiatry. 419 Park Avenue, South. New York, New York. 1970.

This Committee on Aging monograph deals with the type and quality of services, financial aspects of care and training and research.

Verwoerdt, Adriaan. Clinical Geropsychiatry. Williams and Wilkins. Baltimore, Maryland. 1976.

A guide to understanding the psychopathology of aging, which also suggests a treatment approach related to causes of symptoms associated with aging.

von Hahn, H. P. (Editor). Practical Geriatrics. S. Karger. Basel. Switzerland. 1975.

Twenty-three internationally recognized specialists discuss the diagnosis, management, and treatment of the most frequently encountered diseases of the elderly. This book is meant to assist the general practitioner confronted with an increasing number of geriatric patients.

Walford, R. L., et al. The Relation of Aging to Immunity. MSS Information Corporation. New York, New York. 1973.

A consideration of the immunological effects of aging with respect to disease states, autoimmunity, and immunologic tolerance.

Weeks, H. Ashley, and Darsky, Benjamin J. The Urban Aged: Race and Medical Care. School of Public Health. Bureau of Public Health Economics. Research Series No. 14. University of Michigan. Ann Arbor, Michigan. 1968.

Report on a study of the differential use of health services by several subgroups of the aged, with particular attention to the urban Negro aged. The differences in need for, use of, and out-of-pocket expenditures for medical care are considered.

Whitehead, J. A. In the Service of Old Age. Penguin Books, Inc. Baltimore, Maryland. 1970.

A discussion of the welfare of psychogeriatric patients, including emergency service, in-patient service, and a chapter on Severalls Hospital and its psychogeriatric unit.

_______________. Psychiatric Disorders in Old Age: A Handbook for the Clinical Team. Springer Publishing Company. New York, New York. 1974.

The American edition of a British handbook written for psychogeriatric practitioners. Specific treatment methodologies are defined, with case histories used as illustrative materials.

Willington, F. L. (Editor). Incontinence in the Elderly. Academic Press. New York, New York. 1976.

The coverage of this subject includes basic information concerning causes and prevalence, treatments and patient management designed to preserve continence.

Wolff, Kurt. Geriatric Psychiatry. Charles C. Thomas. Springfield, Illinois. 1963.

Description of a treatment, care and rehabilitation approach to emotionally disturbed older persons. An older publication, but one that still has value.

Woodford-Williams, E., and Exton-Smith, A. N. (Editors). Intensive Course in Geriatrics for General Practitioners. S. Karger. New York, New York. 1967.

Although not a recent book, it has value for interested physicians.

Wrench, G. T. The Wheel of Health. Schocken Press. New York, New York. 1972.

A physician emphasizes the need to study healthy rather than ill people, to determine why certain societies are not as prone to disease. He gives special attention to the Hunza society and its longevity.

U. S. GOVERNMENT PUBLICATIONS

Alternatives to Nursing Home Care: A Proposal. Prepared for use by the United States Senate Special Committee on Aging by Staff Specialists at the Levinson Gerontoloigical Policy Institute. Brandeis University. Waltham, Massachusetts. Superintendent of Documents. U. S. Government Printing Office. Washington, D. C. October, 1971.

Anderson, Thomas E., and Blank, Marie L. NIMH Research on the Mental Health of the Aging. Department of Health, Education and Welfare. Publication No. (HSM) 72-9133. Superintendent of Documents. U. S. Government Printing Office. Washington, D. C. 1972.

Barriers to Health Care for Older Americans. Special Committee on Aging. Subcommittee on Health of the Elderly. United States Senate. Ninety-third Congress. First Session. Superintendent of Documents. U. S. Government Printing Office. Washington, D. C. 1973.

Characteristics of Patients Treated by Podiatrists: United States 1970. National Center for Health Statistics. DHEW Publication No. (HRA) 75-1089. Superintendent of Documents. U. S. Government Printing Office. Washington, D. C. 1971.

Chinn, Austin B., et al. Physical and Mental Health: Background Issues. White House Conference on Aging. Superintendent of Documents. U. S. Government Printing Office. Washington, D. C. 1971.

________________ (Editor). Working With Older People: A Guide to Practice. Vol. IV. Clinical Aspects of Aging. PHS Publication No. 1459. Superintendent of Documents. U. S. Government Printing Office. Washington, D. C. 1971.

Convalescence at Home Following Hospitalization Among Persons 55 Years of Age and Older, United States. July 1966-June 1967. National Center for Health Statistics. U. S. Department of Health, Education and Welfare. DHEW Publication No. (HSM) 72-1029. Superintendent of Documents. U. S. Government Printing Office. Washington, D. C. 1971.

Cooper, Barbara S., and Piro, Paula A. Age Differences in Medical Care Spending: Fiscal Year 1973. Social Security Administration. U. S. Department of Health, Education and Welfare. DHEW Publication No. (SSA) 74-11701. Superintendent of Documents. U. S. Government Printing Office. Washington, D. C. 1974.

Granick, Samuel, and Patterson, Robert D. Human Aging II: An Eleven-Year Followup Biomedical and Behavioral Study. U. S. Department of Health, Education and Welfare. National Institute of Mental Health. DHEW Publication No. (HSM) 71-9037. Rockville, Maryland. 1971.

Health Care Strategies. White House Conference on Aging. Superintendent of Documents. U. S. Government Printing Office. Washington, D. C. 1972.

Hearing Aids and the Older American. Subcommittee on Consumer Interests of the Elderly. United States Senate Special Committee on Aging. Ninety-third Congress. First Session. Superintendent of Documents. U. S. Government Printing Office. Washington, D. C. 1974.

Mental Health and the Elderly. Joint Hearing Before the Subcommittee on Long-Term Care and the Subcommittee on Health of the Elderly of the Special Committee on Aging. United States Senate. Ninety-fourth Congress. First Session. September 29, 1975. Superintendent of Documents. U. S. Government Printing Office. Washington, D. C. 1976.

Mental Health Care and the Elderly: Shortcomings in Public Policy. A Report by the Special Committee on Aging. United States Senate. Superintendent of Documents. U. S. Government Printing Office. Washington, D. C. 1971.

Namey, Christy, and Wilson, Ronald W. Age Patterns in Medical Care, Illness, and Disability: United States, 1968-1969. Division of Health Interview Statistics. National Center for Health Services Research and Development. U. S. Department of Health, Education and Welfare. DHEW Publication No. (HSM) 72-1026. Superintendent of Documents. U. S. Government Printing Office. Washington, D. C. 1972.

New Perspectives in Health Care for Older Americans. Report of Subcommittee on Health and Long Term Care, House Select Committee on Aging. Ninety-fourth Congress. Superintendent of Documents. U. S. Government Printing Office. Washington, D. C. 1976.

Progress Report on Regional Medical Programs for Heart Disease, Cancer, Stroke, and Related Disease. Maryland: Division of Regional Medical Programs. Health Services and Mental Health Administration and Department of Health, Education and Welfare. Superintendent of Documents. U. S. Government Printing Office. Washington, D. C. 1969.

Ryan, Kenneth J., and Gibson, Don C. Menopause and Aging. U. S. Department of Health, Education and Welfare. National Institute of Health. Publication No. 73-319. Superintendent of Documents. U.S. Government Printing Office. Washington, D. C. 1973.

Atchley, Robert C., and Seltzer, Mildred M. Developing Educational Programs in the Field of Aging. Scripps Foundation Gerontology Center. Miami University. Oxford, Ohio. 1974.

This source provides course outlines, a bibliography of gerontological texts, as well as guidance in establishing field work opportunities.

Comprehensive Bibliography on Educational Gerontology, A. Institute of Gerontology. University of Michigan-Wayne State University. Ann Arbor, Michigan. 1971.

A list of publications and materials in 20 separate areas of educational gerontology and training.

Davis, Richard, H., et al (Editors). The Role of Institutions of Higher Learning in the Study of Aging. Ethel Percy Andrus Gerontology Center. University of Southern California. Los Angeles, California. 1973.

A collection of papers on gerontology as it relates to the changing role of education in society, the place of gerontology in higher education, and the multidisciplinary aspects of gerontology education.

Deichman, E. S., and O'Kane, C. P. (Editors). Working with the Elderly: A Training Manual. D. O. K. Publishers, Inc. Buffalo, New York. 1975.

A manual emphasizing concepts about the aging and the importance of activity programs that emphasize remotivation and rehabilitation. Covers both physical and psychological aspects from points of view of physicians, nurses, therapists, social workers and activity directors.

Delivery and Administration of Services for the Elderly. University of Southern California. Commission on Aging. Sacramento, California. 1970.

Materials designed to aid in teaching and studying the delivery and administration of services to the aged.

Ernst, Marvin, and Shore, Herbert. _Sensitizing People to the Process of Aging: The In-Service Educator's Guide._ Center for Studies in Aging. School of Community Service. North Texas University. Denton, Texas. 1975.

A guide for in-service instructors to use in enhancing awareness of sensory changes in older persons.

Gentry, W. Doyle (Editor). Geropsychology: _A Model of Training and Clinical Service._ Ballinger Publishing Company. Cambridge, Massachusetts. 1975.

Description of the role of applied clinical psychology in care of the aged; curriculum for training; psychological treatment; issues to be considered in psychological diagnosis; and the application of research to clinical practice.

Hansen, Gary D., et al. _Decade for Action in Gerontology and Geriatric Care: Education-Research-Services-Facilities: Long Range Plan 1966-1976._ Mt. Angel College. Mt. Angel, Oregon. 1966.

Title Self explanatory.

Kushner, Rose E., and Bunch, Marion E. (Editors). _Graduate Education in Aging Within the Social Sciences._ Division of Gerontology. University of Mighican. Ann Arbor, Michigan. 1967.

A guide for universities and other training institutions in organizing and implementing graduate programs of education in social gerontology.

Media Resources: A Comprehensive Listing. Resources in Aging. Institute of Gerontology. University of Michigan. Ann Arbor, Michigan. 1974.

A 60-page guide which lists and describes more than 250 films, filmstrips, feature films, slides, transparencies, and audio tapes relating to aging.

Pearlman, Lou W., et al. _Social Casework - Field Work Training in a Geriatric Institutional Study: Review of a Five-Year Experiment_. Public Welfare Project on Aging. American Public Welfare Association. Chicago, Illinois. October, 1968.

Description of a student training program developed by the School of Social Service Administration, the University of Chicago, which offered field work in the Drexel Home for the Aged.

Piluras, Chris. _How to Plan Better Meetings and Training Programs._ Senior Opportunities and Services. Technical Assistance Monograph No. 10. National Council on the Aging. Washington, D. C. 1972.

A summary and review of some of the more popular training techniques used by educators and trainers in working with the aged.

Powers, Edward A., and Golinvaux, J. P. _The Aged in an Affluent Society: A Resource Book_. Cooperative Extension Service. Iowa State University. Ames, Iowa. 1972.

An aid to extension service personnel in development of educational and program activities, etc., in the field of aging.

Psycho-Social Needs of the Aged: Selected Papers, The. Ethel Percy Andrus Gerontology Center. University of Southern California. Los Angeles, California. 1973.

A collection of edited papers which have been delivered at seminars and institutes sponsored by the Gerontology Center to train those who provide services to the elderly. There are three main divisions: Needs, Care, and Training.

Report on the Proceedings of the First and Second Symposia on Education, Training and Aging, A. New England Center for Continuing Education. Durham, New Hampshire. 1975.

A compilation of keynote addresses and major presentations given at two regional sumposia. Topics include: role and function in old age, education, work, retirement.

Rosencranz, Howard A. (Editor). Pre-Retirement Education: A Manual for Conference Leaders. Program in Gerontology, University of Connecticut. Storrs, Connecticut. 1975.

Written for use in Connecticut, two of the four sections of the manual, which cover pre-retirement education program organization and topics to be encompassed, have general applicability.

Saul, Shura. Aging: An Album of People Growing Old. John Wiley & Sons, Inc. New York, New York. 1974.

A combination of recent research findings and authentic vignettes of people growing old; aimed at improvement of the emotional and cognitive skills of those in the service professions.

Schwartz, Arthur, and Burnside, Irene Mortenson. Model Continuing Education Program: Psychosocial Care in Nursing Homes. Ethel Percy Andrus Gerontology Center. University of Southern California. Los Angeles, California. 1974.

A brief report and a training manual for use with key personnel in long term care facilities. The Premise is that attitudinal and behavioral changes in leadership personnel will affect the total institution.

Schwartz, Beverly (Editor). Utilization of College Resources in Gerontology: A Program Guide. Montclair State College. Department of Adult Continuing Education. Upper Montclair, New Jersey. 1976.

Guidelines for use by four year colleges in implementing gerontology education programs providing educational and training services to community agencies serving the aged and facilitating college program and services for older adults.

U. S. GOVERNMENT PUBLICATIONS

Homemaker Health Aide Service Training Manual. DHEW Publication No. (OHD) 74-20103. Homemaker Health Aide Service of the National Capital Area, Inc. Administration on Aging. Department of Health, Education and Welfare. Washington, D. C. (N.D.)

Mental Health Continuing Education Programs for Long-Term Care Providers. National Institute of Mental Health. Public Health Service. U. S. Department of Health, Education and Welfare. Superintendent of Documents. U. S. Government Printing Office. Washington, D. C. 1975.

Mental Health: Principles and Training Techniques in Nursing Home Care. U. S. Department of Health, Education and Welfare. Health Services and Mental Health Administration. National Institute of Mental Health. DHEW Publication No. (HSM) 73-9046. Superintendent of Documents. U. S. Government Printing Office. Washington, D. C. 1972.

National Directory of Educational Programs in Gerontology. The Association for Gerontology on Higher Education. Superintendent of Documents. U. S. Government Printing Office. Washington, D. C. or The National Clearinghouse on Aging. Administration on Aging. Washington, D. C. 1976.

Rich, Thomas A., and Gilmore, Alden S. Basic Concepts of Aging: A Programmed Manual. U. S. Department of Health, Education and Welfare. AOA Publication No. 274. Superintendent of Documents. U. S. Government Printing Office. Washington, D. C. 1969.

Training in Social Gerontology and Its Application: A Suggested University Curriculum. U. S. Office on Aging. Division of Research and Training. Superintendent of Documents. U. S. Government Printing Office. Washington, D. C. 1965.

Training Needs in Gerontology. Hearing before the Special Committee on Aging. United States Senate. Ninety-Fourth Congress. March, 1975. U. S. Government Printing Office. Washington, D. C. 1975.

Training Needs in Gerontology. Special Committee on Aging. United States Senate. Ninety-Third Congress. First Session. Superintendent of Documents. U. S. Government Printing Office. Washington, D. C. 1973.

Working With Older People: A Guide to Practice. Volume I: The Practitioner and the Elderly. Public Health Service. Publication No. 1459. Superintendent of Documents. U. S. Government Printing Office. Washington, D. C. 1966.

HEALTH MAINTENANCE AND PREVENTIVE CARE

Anderson, W. Ferguson. Practical Management of the Elderly. Second Edition. Blackwell Scientific Publications. Oxford, England. 1971.

Survey of the medical, psychological and social problems of the aged; offers preventive measures for planning to meet their needs.

Brunner, D., and Jokl, E. (Editors). Physical Activity and Aging: With Special Reference to the Effect of Exercise and Training on the Natural History of Arteriosclerotic Heart Disease. University Park Press. Baltimore, Maryland. 1970.

Treatise on the importance of physical exercise in reducing skeletal deterioration in the aging process.

Duke, C. E. How to be Young at Sixty. Exposition Press. Hicksville, New York. 1975.

Suggestions for maintenance of youthfulness into old age that center around such areas as exercise, diet, meditation, humor.

Geba, Bruno. Vitality Training for Older Adults: A Positive Approach to Growing Old. Random House. New York, New York. 1974.

Vitality training is presented as a tool for changing defeatist attitudes towards old age by understanding and adaptation.

Harris, Raymond, et al (Editors). Guide to Fitness After Fifty. Plenum Press. New York, New York. 1976.

Presentation of results from research and practice promoting physical activity programs to enrich the lives of those over 50.

Health Maintenance Service for the Older Adult, A. National Council on the Aging. Washington, D. C. 1972.

Description of a coordinate neighborhood health services program to provide essential care for the aged poor.

Hyachovec, J. P. Keeping Young and Living Longer: How to Stay Active and Healthy Past 100. Sherbourne Press. Los Angeles, California. 1972.

Discussion of the potential which each person has to live past 100 years. Suggestions are given for achieving this.

Kahn, Samuel. Essays on Longevity. Philosophical Library, Inc. New York, New York. 1974.

A physician writes on a variety of topics related to maintenance of physical and psychological health. Emphasizes the positive correlation between boredom and fatigue.

King, Frances, and Herzig, William F. Golden Age Exercises. Crown Publishers. New York, New York. 1968.

Descriptions of use-tested exercises given by a physical therapist for keeping fit and for feeling mentally and physically strong.

McConnell, Grace B. Multiphasic Health Screening for the Senior Population. Senior Citizens, Inc. 1801 Broadway. Nashville, Tennessee. 1974.

Report on a multiphasic health screening project in Nashville, Tennessee.

Pfeiffer, Eric (Editor). Alternatives to Institutional Care for Older Americans: Practices and Planning. Center for the Study of Aging and Human Development. Duke University. Durham, North Carolina. 1973.

Report of a national conference held at Duke University in 1972. Areas explored are: designing systems of care; planning at all governmental levels; training planners and practitioners; and innovative approaches.

________________________, Multidimensional Functional Assessment: The OARS Methodology: A Manual. Duke University. Durham, North Carolina. 1975.

A compilation of rationales, methodologies and techniques for assessment of functional levels with emphasis upon older adults, including physical and mental health, economic and social resources.

Planning Health Services. Syracuse University School of Social Work. Senior Opportunities and Services, Technical Assistance Monograph No. 8. National Council on the Aging. Washington, D. C. 1971.

A monograph on basic issues and programs pertaining to health care.

Reynolds, Frank W., and Barsam, Paul C. Adult Health: Services for Chronically Ill and Aged. The Macmillan Company. New York, New York. 1967.

This volume is divided into four parts: Components of an Adult Health Program; Supporting Services; Categorical and Chronic Disease Control Programs; and Federal and State Programs and Financing of Costs.

Rossman, Isadore (Editor). Clinical Geriatrics. J. B. Lippincott Company. Philadelphia, Pennsylvania. 1971.

Authoritative, practical help in care and guidance of normal aging people; the prevention of some disorders; and description of expert management of the geriatric patient.

Rothenberg, Robert E. Health in the Later Years. The New American Library of World Literature. New York, New York. 1970.

Attention is given to defining and describing disabilities that are prevalent in later life and coping with these for better health in old age.

Schwartz, Arthur N. (Editor). Assessment and Therapy in Aging. The Ethel Percy Andrus Gerontology Center. University of Southern California. Los Angeles, California. 1975.

Subjects covered emphasize the importance of diagnostic assessment and health maintenance therapy.

Stonecypher, D. D. Getting Older and Staying Young: A Doctor's Prescription for Continuing Vitality in Later Life. W. W. Norton. New York, New York. 1974.

Explanation of the aging process and a prescription for continuing vitality in later life.

Thostenson, George C. To Your Good Health - After 50. Field Enterprizes, Inc. Fawcett Publishing Corporation. Rockville, Maryland. 1972.

Written for older persons, a guide to understanding aging changes, health problems and care.

Tiven, Marjorie Bloomberg. Health Maintenance Programs in Senior Centers. The National Council on the Aging. Washington, D. C. 1973.

An examination of preventive health programs in Senior Center services, their strengths and development. Includes discussion on working with older minority groups and use of community resources.

Wassersug, Joseph D. How to be Healthy and Happy After Sixty. Abelard-Schuman. New York, New York. 1966.

A discussion of health maintenance for mind and body.

Winter, Ruth. Ageless Aging: How Science is Winning the Battle to Help You Extend Your Healthy and Productive Years. Crown Publishers, Inc. New York, New York. 1973.

A book which discusses ways to increase vigor and prolong youthfulness as the result of scientific advances already being made.

U. S. GOVERNMENT PUBLICATIONS

Adult Day Facilities for Treatment, Health Care, and Related Services. Special Committee on Aging. U. S. Senate. U. S. Government Printing Office. Washington, D. C. 1976.

Adult Physical Fitness: A Program for Men and Women. President's Council on Physical Fitness. U. S. Government Printing Office. Washington, D. C. 1973.

Air Pollution Advice for Elderly. Environmental Protection Agency. Superintendent of Documents. U. S. Government Printing Office. Washington, D. C. 1972.

Barriers to Health Care for Older Americans. Subcommittee on Health of the Elderly. Special Committee on Aging. Ninety-third Congress. First Session. U. S. Senate. Superintendent of Documents. U. S. Government Printing Office. Washington, D. C. 1973.

Fitness Challenge in the Later Years, The. U. S. Department of Health, Education and Welfare. Social and Rehabilitation Service. Administration on Aging. Superintendent of Documents. U. S. Government Printing Office. Washington, D. C. 1968.

Health In the Later Years of Life. U. S. Department of Health, Education and Welfare. Public Health Service. Publication No. 1722-0178. Health Services and Mental Health Administration. National Center for Health Statistics. Superintendent of Documents. U. S. Government Printing Office. Washington, D. C. October, 1971.

Mental Health and the Elderly. Joint Hearing Before the Subcommittee on Long-Term Care and the Subcommittee on Health of the Elderly. Senate Special Committee on Aging. Superintendent of Documents. U. S. Government Printing Office. Washington, D. C. 1975.

Office Evaluation of the Aging Patient. U. S. Department of Health, Education, and Welfare. Public Health Service. Publication No. 1513. Superintendent of Documents. U. S. Government Printing Office. Washington, D. C. August, 1966.

Portraits in Community Health: The Dexter Manor Story. U. S. Department of Health, Education, and Welfare. Public Health Service. Publication No. 1344-3. Superintendent of Documents. U. S. Government Printing Office. Washington, D. C. October, 1966.

LIVING ARRANGEMENTS AND HOUSING

Alternatives to Institutional Care. National Council on the Aging. Washington, D. C. Revised periodically.

An annotated bibliography.

Atchley, Robert, and Byerts, Thomas O. (Editors). _Rural Environments and Aging_. Gerontological Society. Washington, D. C. 1975.

Compilation of conference papers on a variety of related topics.

Barker, Michael B. _California Retirement Communities_. Center for Real Estate and Urban Economics. Institute of Urban and Regional Development. University of California. Berkeley, California. 1966. (Special Report No. 2)

A review of the organizational and management aspects of two retirement communities and a look at the relationships between these communities and their respective municipal corporations.

Beyer, Glenn H., and Nierstrasz, F. H. J. _Housing the Aged in Western Countries: Programs, Dwellings, Homes and Geriatric Facilities_. American Elsevier. New York, New York. 1967.

A comparative analysis of housing in Western countries.

Building Better: _A Survey of Ontario Homes for the Aged as Viewed by Residents and an Independent Group of Senior Citizens_. Two Volumes, Looseleaf. Associated Senior Executives of Canada, Ltd. Toronto, Ontario, Canada. 1974.

Report on a survey of residents in homes for the aged which served as a basis for extensive recommendations.

Burgess, Ernest W. (Editor). _Retirement Villages_. Division of Gerontology. The University of Michigan. Ann Arbor, Michigan. 1961.

Reports of a Conference on Retirement Villages sponsored by the American Society of the Aged. Despite its age, this book is still considered a worthwhile reference.

Byerts, Thomas O. (Editor). Environmental Research and Aging: Report From an Interdisciplinary Research Development Conference. The Gerontological Society. Washington, D. C. 1974.

A collection of papers which suggest ways in which human factor engineering can be used to design housing to meet the protective physical environmental needs of the aged.

_________________ (Editor). Housing and Environment for the Elderly. Gerontological Society. Washington, D. C. 1974.

Complete proceedings of the Gerontological Society's working Conference on Behavioral Research Utilization and Environmental Policy held in San Juan, Puerto Rico, December 16-20, 1971.

_________________ (Editor). Residential Environments for the Functionally Disabled. Gerontological Society. Washington, D. C. 1975.

A final report on the project to assess individual capacity and environmental adequacy. Includes population assessment and environmental evaluation, among other topics. Applicable to the aged as well as to others.

_________________ (Editor). "The City: A Viable Environment for the Elderly?" The Gerontologist. Vol. 15. February, 1975.

Reports from a symposium which attempted to bring together research findings regarding the city as a place for the aged to live.

Carp, Frances M. A Future for the Aged: Victoria Plaza and Its Residents. University of Texas Press. Austin, Texas. 1966.

A comprehensive report on psycho-social aspects of public housing for the elderly, based on a study in San Antonio, Texas.

Christison, James A. Emphasis on Living. Judson Press. Valley Forge, Pennsylvania. 1970.

Living rather than housing is emphasized in this manual based upon the experiences of the American Home Mission Societies' retirement housing program. Simply written guidelines for organizing, planning, financing, operating, and administering a retirement housing center.

Coggeshall, John H. Management of Retirement Homes and Long Term Care Facilities. The C. V. Mosby Company. St. Louis. Missouri. 1973.

A book dealing with the administration and management of facilities providing housing for the elderly and for long term care.

Davis, Richard H. (Editor). Housing for the Elderly. Ethel Percy Andrus Gerontology Center. University of Southern California. Los Angeles, California. 1973.

A collection of papers presented at a career development institute for sponsors, owners, and administrators of congregate housing facilities for the aged; offers pertinent information and ideas for facility planning and services.

__________________, et al (Editors). Non-Profit Homes for the Aging: Planning, Development, and Programming. Ethel Percy Andrus Gerontology Center. University of Souther California. Los Angeles, California. 1973.

Specific information, techniques, and reference materials to aid sponsors and developers in initial development, redevelopment, or expansion of housing facilities and services for the aged.

Directory of Jewish Homes for the Aged in U. S. and Canada. National Association of Jewish Homes for the Aged. Dallas, Texas. (Updated periodically).

Summary of licensure, accreditation, finances, staff, social services, leisure time programs, medical facilities, building programs, ages of residents, and board of directors of the Jewish Homes for the Aged.

Eisdorfer, Carl (Editor). Environments and Aging: Concepts and Issues. The Gerontological Society. Washington, D. C. 1976.

This text covers: identification of the elderly, their adaptation to their environment, research and design application and education.

Eisdorfer, Carl, et al (Editors). *Housing and Environment Project: Final Report, 1971-1975*. Gerontological Society. Washington, D. C. 1976.

The findings from a study covering: research in environments and aging, housing policies, design and the building field, and accommodations for research and design development.

Frush, James, and Eschenbach, Benson. *The Retirement Residence: An Analysis of the Architecture and Management of Life-Care Housing*. Charles C. Thomas. Springfield, Illinois. 1968.

A discussion of design construction, and operation of a retirement home as an adequate environment for the aged, and consideration of economic feasibility determinants.

Furniture Requirements for Older People. The National Council on the Aging, Inc. Washington, D. C. 1963.

A description of basic considerations in the designing of furniture for the aged. An older publication still available.

Gelwicks, Louis E., and Byerts, Thomas O. *Living Arrangements of Older People*. University of Southern California Gerontology Center. Los Angeles, California. 1969.

A discussion of older people's needs and how they might be served in the living environment.

__________, and Newcomer, Robert J. *Planning, Environment and the Older Person*. National Council on the Aging. Washington, D. C. 1973.

An examination of the integral relationships between living arrangements and services which affect the quality of life for the elderly.

__________. *Planning House Environments for the Elderly*. National Council on the Aging. Washington, D. C. 1974.

Quoting the Executive Director of NCOA, this book was designed as a tool for those concerned with planning buildings and managing housing for the aged. Explicit guidelines are given for planning, furnishing, and equipping housing for the elderly.

Green, Isaac, et al. Housing for the Elderly: The Development and Design Process. Van Nostrand Reinhold. New York, New York. 1975.

A guide to alternatives in housing which includes independent living as well as institutions; relates housing needs to physical, psychological and social needs of the aged.

Gubrium, Jaber F. (Editor). Late Life: Communities and Environmental Policy. Charles C. Thomas. Springfield, Illinois. 1975.

A collection of original papers examining the impact of the social environment upon older adults. Environmental policy issues are treated as well as different types of environment, such as age integrated and age segregated communities.

Hochschild, Arlie Russell. The Unexpected Community. Prentice-Hall. Englewood Cliffs, New Jersey. 1973.

Examination of the life style for a group of old people living in a small apartment building in the San Francisco Bay area.

Holter, Paul. Guide to Retirement Living. Rand McNally and Company. New York, New York.

Text includes basic preparation, retirement living decisions and types of choices. There is an extensive list of retirement facilities in the United States.

Housing and Living Arrangements for Older People. National Council on the Aging. Washington, D. C. (Revised periodically.)

An annotated bibliography.

Housing for the Elderly Development Process. The Michigan State Housing Development Authority. Lansing, Michigan. 1974.

Guidelines for housing design for the elderly from site selection through construction.

"Housing for the Elderly - A Symposium Presented at the 21st Annual Meeting of the Gerontological Society." The Gerontologist. Vol. 9, No. 1. Gerontological Society. Washington, D. C. Spring, 1969.

Issue devoted to concerns in housing as presented in papers at the 21st Annual Meeting of the Gerontological Society.

Housing the Low-Income Elderly. Richmond Redevelopment and Housing Authority. Richmond, Virginia. Spetember, 1974.

A report concerned with the special housing needs of the elderly of Richmond, Virginia, but one which has more general applicability as it includes such topics as problems of low-income elderly and design of low-income housing for the elderly.

Improving the Living Environment of the Elderly Poor. Syracuse University School of Social Work. Prepared by Senior Opportunities and Services. Technical Assistance Monograph No. 7. National Council on the Aging. Washington, D. C. 1971.

A monograph written for Community Action Agencies to point out the kinds of programs which might improve the environment of the aged.

Invisible Elderly, The. Proceedings of Conference on "Single Room Only Elderly." St. Louis University. 1975. Institute of Applied Gerontology. St. Louis University. St. Louis, Missouri. 1976.

The topics include the need to identify the elderly who live in hotels and rooming houses, to understand their characteristics and needs, their relationship to public policy, and the results of research in this area.

Jacobs, Jerry. Older Persons and Retirement Communities. Charles C. Thomas. Springfield, Illinois. 1975.

The pros and cons of segregated living for older persons are discussed.

Johnson, Sheila K. Idle Haven: Community Building Among the Working-Class Retired. University of California Press. Berkeley, California. 1971.

A descriptive study of life in a mobile home park for the aged.

Joyce, David, et al. The Social Functioning of the Disloged Elderly: A Study of Post-Relocation Assistance. Institute for Environmental Studies. University of Pennsylvania. Philadelphia, Pennsylvania. 1966.

Ways to overcome difficulties faced by elderly people in re-establishing social ties in a new neighborhood.

Kenover, John. Micah: A Case Study In Housing Rehabilitation Through Nonprofit Sponsorship. Department of Community Affairs. Providence, Rhode Island. 1969.

A study which points out the necessity of social as well as physical programs in solving housing problems in urban areas.

Kessler, Judy. Cohesiveness and Aging: An Empirical Test. University of Nebraska. Center for Urban Affairs. Omaha, Nebraska. 1969.

Study of interaction patterns among elderly residents in public housing which finds no support for the disengagement theory; should be helpful to those planning housing for the aged.

Koncelik, Joseph A. Considerate Design and the Aging: Review Article With a Selected and Annotated Bibliography. Council of Planning Libraries. Monticello, Illinois. 1972.

A review of literature specifically related to design of both products and physical environment for older persons.

_________________, and Byerts, Thomas O. (Editors). Design and Development of Housing Products for the Elderly. Gerontological Society. Washington, D. C. 1975.

Report on a 1974 conference of engineers, industrial designers, manufacturers and researchers. Topics covered are furniture and interior design, hardware, appliances.

Lange, John D. *Local Action Programs: Housing for Older Americans.* National Retired Teachers Association and American Association of Retired Persons. 1909 K Street, N. W. Washington, D. C. 1974.

A monograph prepared for the National Forum on Aging for Local Government Officials to provide community leaders with general information regarding the housing needs of the elderly and the programs and resources available to meet their needs.

Lawton, M. Powell. *Planning and Managing Housing for the Elderly.* John Wiley and Sons. New York, New York. 1975.

This book offers an introduction to the field of housing for the aged including extent of needs, and the planning and administration of such facilities. Examines public and private housing programs, and covers a number of socio-economic aspects of housing for the aged.

Lohmann, Roger, and Lohmann, Nancy. *Medicare, Medicaid and Geriatric Residential Environments.* American Rehabilitation Foundation. Minneapolic, Minnesota. 1971.

An analysis of housing developments for the aged in the 1960's.

Lowman, Edward W., and Klinger, Judith L. *Aids to Independent Living.* McGraw-Hill Book Company. New York, New York. 1969.

Title self explanatory. Value not limited to older persons.

May, E. E., et al. *Independent Living for the Handicapped and the Elderly.* Houghton-Mifflin Company. Boston, Massachusetts. 1975.

A practical guide to solutions to many of the problems that confront handicapped and elderly persons. Includes suggestions for independent living and for recreation and travel; appendices give sources of information and aid.

McClure, Ethel. *More Than a Roof: The Development of Minnesota Poor Farms and Homes for the Aged.* Minnesota Historical Society. St. Paul, Minnesota. 1968.

Historical account of the development of homes for the aged in Minnesota, and an analysis of change and trends in care of Minnesota's aged from 1850 to 1960.

McGuire, Marie C. Design of Housing for the Elderly: A Checklist. National Association of Housing and Redevelopment Officials. Publication No. N560. Washington, D. C. October, 1972.

A checklist of features which should be incorporated into housing for the aged.

McRae, John. Elderly in the Environment: Northern Europe. Center for Gerontological Studies and Programs. University of Florida. Gainesville, Florida. 1976.

An architect studied in Holland, Denmark, Norway, Finland and Sweden to understand the needs of the elderly there to determine how needs were interpreted by housing and social planning, and to interpret the resulting physical environments.

Management of Public Housing for the Elderly: Background Readings. National Association for Housing and Redevelopment Officials. Washington, D. C. 1965.

A collection of authoritative papers devoted to characteristics of low-income elderly for use by housing management staffs.

Manard, Barbara B., et al. Old Age Institutions. Lexington Books. Lexington, Maine. 1975.

A fact finding report on nursing homes and housing for the aged in the United States. Consideration is given to the impact of federal subsidies and regulations on old-age institutions in this country.

Mattice, Royal. Florida Retirement Hotels: Functions, Services and Relations. Florida Commission on Aging. Tallahassee, Florida. 1968.

Investigation of retirement hotels and their residents, the services available and those needed.

Musson, Nouverre. The National Directory of Retirement Residences: Best Places to Live When You Retire. Frederick Fell Publishers. New York, New York. 1973.

Discussion of the needs of retirees; provides information on residences available to them in the United States, and contains a list of over 1,000 retirement residences.

Niebanck, Paul L., and Yessian, Mark. Relocation in Urban Planning: From Obstacle to Opportunity. University of Pennsylvania Press. .Philadephia, Pennsylvania. 1968.

A primary emphasis is given to suggestions and recommendations related to growing problems of displaced elderly persons in American cities. Elderly housing and its adaptive environment is offered as a support to maintaining independence.

On-Site Housing Manager's Resource Book: Housing for the Elderly, The. National Center for Housing Management, Inc. Washington, D. C.

A resource book concerned with knowledge needs and problems inherent in management of housing for the aged. All types of housing, including Federal Housing, are covered. A large portion of the book is devoted to how to cope with specific areas of management.

Pastalan, Leon A., and Carson, Daniel H. (Editors). Spatial Behavior of Older People. University of Michigan-Wayne State University Institute of Gerontology. Ann Arbor, Michigan. 1970.

A collection of papers focusing on the utilization of space and spatial arrangements in residential settings for the elderly.

Patterns for Progress. Institute on Housing for the Aged. Central Bureau for the Jewish Aged. New York, New York. 1968.

Insight into ways of working with government agencies in order to facilitate implementation of existing housing legislation.

Pearce, Donn. Dying in the Sun. Charterhouse. New York, New York. 1974.

A description of old people living out their lives in a retirement setting in Florida. Emphasis in upon negative factors.

Pfeiffer, Eric (Editor). National Conference on Alternatives to Institutional Care for Older Americans. Duke University Press. Durham, North Carolina. 1973.

Proceedings of the conference held at Duke University, which cover a diversity of topics related to avoidance of institutionalization for older persons.

Rabinowitz, Dorothy, and Nielson, Yedida. Home Life: A Story of Old Age. The Macmillan Company. New York, New York. 1971.

Description of life in two homes for the aged; fiction based upon real experiences.

Regnier, Victor (Editor). Environmental Concerns of the Aged. University of Southern California. Los Angeles, California. 1976.

Consideration is given to the needs and problems related to housing which older persons themselves have recognized.

________________________. Environmental Planning for the Elderly. The Ethel Percy Andrus Gerontology Center. University of Southern California. Los Angeles, California. 1975.

A bibliography.

Relocation Reports. Institute of Gerontology. The University of Michigan-Wayne State University. Ann Arbor, Michigan.

A series of reports on research on relocation of sick elderly people. Attention is focused on preparing the elderly for relocation, psychological and environmental factors in relocation, effects of relocation upon the lives of the elderly, and implications of these effects for policy-making. Titles of the three reports are as follows: 1. Work in Progress, 2. Death and Survival, and 3. Preparation for Relocation.

Senior Advisory Service for Public Housing Tenants: Report and Recommendations to the Committee on Aging and the Committee on Housing and Urban Development. Community Service Society of New York. New York, New York. 1969.

A study of persons living in public housing which examines needed health services, psychological adjustments, activities and social relationships. Includes a look at the involvement of elderly persons in meeting some of these needs.

Shore, Herbert, and the Staff of Golden Acres. Adventures in Group Living. Dallas Home for the Jewish Aged. Dallas, Texas. 1972.

Selected writings related to philosophy on aging, institutional care, and social and institutional services.

Silverstone, Barbara M. Establishing Resident Councils. Federation of Protestant Welfare Agencies, Division on Aging. New York, New York. 1974.

Guidelines for residents and administrators desiring to organize or strengthen resident councils in residential facilities for the elderly.

Snyder, Lorraine Hiatt. The Environmental Challenge and the Aging Individual. Council of Planning Librarians. Monticello, Illinois. 1972.

A review of reference materials dealing with environmental effects upon older persons. Includes a 14-page bibliography.

Steinfeld, Edward (Project Director). Barrier-Free Design for the Elderly and the Disabled (Parts 1-3). All-University Gerontology Center and Center for Instructional Development. Syracuse University. Syracuse, New York. 1975.

Not restricted to the aged, this volume discusses the need for elimination of environmental hazards imposed by physical limitations.

Stevens, Joyce. Loners, Losers and Lovers: Elderly Tenants in a Slum Hotel. University of Washington Press. Seattle, Washington. 1976.

A book dealing with the socio-psychological ramifications of hotel housing, and the problems inherent in limitations imposed.

Walkley, Rosabelle Price, et al. Retirement Housing in California. Diablo Press. Berkeley, California. 1966.

Discussion of retirement housing construction, site locations, sponsorship, costs and financial arrangements, programs and services available. A study conducted for the UCLA School of Public Health.

Weiss, Joseph Douglas. Better Buildings for the Aged. McGraw-Hill Book Company, Inc. New York, New York. 1969.

A resource on building construction subjects which runs the gamut from residential housing to nursing care facilities; provides illustrations of the broad variety of design and approaches possible to aid in the delivery of services.

Wellar, Barry S., and Graff, Thomas O. Introduction and Selected Bibliography on the Quality of Housing and its Environment. Council of Planning Librarians. Monticello, Illinois. 1972.

References include both methodology and practical aspects of research and of housing development as they pertain to quality of the environment.

Windley, Paul G, et al (Editors). Theory Development in Environment and Aging. Gerontological Society. Washington, D. C. 1975.

Proceedings of a conference in 1974 designed to further understanding of theories and research concerning man and his environment.

Zelver, Alvin. Considerations In Planning Housing for the Elderly. National Council on the Aging. Washington, D. C. 1972.

Information and advice on location and construction of housing and supportive facilities for the aged.

U. S. GOVERNMENT PUBLICATIONS

Adequacy of Federal Response to Housing Needs of Older Americans. Hearing before Subcommittee on Housing for the Elderly, Special Committee on Aging. United States Senate. Ninety-Fourth Congress. First Session. Part 13. U. S. Government Printing Office. Washington, D. C. 1976.

Adequacy of Federal Response to Housing Needs of Older Americans. Subcommittee on Housing for the Elderly. Special Committee on Aging. Ninety-Third Congress. Second Session. United States Senate. Superintendent of Documents. U. S. Government Printing Office. Washington, D. C. 1974.

Alternatives to Institutionalization of Elderly. Subcommittee on Aging and Special Subcommittee on Human Resources. Labor and Public Welfare Committee. United States Senate. Ninety-Third Congress. First Session. Washington, D. C. 1973.

Barrier-Free Environment for the Elderly and the Handicapped, A. Special Committee on Aging. Ninety-Second Congress. First Session. United States Senate. Superintendent of Documents. U. S. Government Printing Office. Washington, D. C. 1972.

"Basic Laws and Authorities on Housing and Urban Development." Revised through January 31, 1971. United States Congress. House of Representatives. Committee on Banking and Currency. Superintendent of Documents. U. S. Government Printing Office. Washington, D. C. 1971.

Built Environment for the Elderly and Handicapped, The. Library and Information Division. Housing and Urban Development Department. Superintendent of Documents. U. S. Government Printing Office. Washington, D. C. 1971. (A bibliography).

Congregate Housing for Older Adults: Assisted Residential Living Combining Shelter and Services. A working paper prepared for Special Committee on Aging. United States Senate. U. S. Government Printing Office. Washington, D. C. November, 1975.

Elderly Housing Overview: HUD's Inaction. Report of House Aging Subcommittee on Housing and Consumer Interests. Ninety-Fourth Congress. Superintendent of Documents. U. S. Government Printing Office. Washington, D. C. 1976.

Examination of Proposed Section 202 Housing Regulations. Hearing Before the Subcommittee on Housing for the Elderly of the Senate Special Committee on Aging. Parts 1 and 2. Superintendent of Documents. U. S. Government Printing Office. Washington, D. C. 1975.

Housing for Elderly: A Status Report. Special Committee on Aging. Ninety-Third Congress. First Session. United States Senate. Superintendent of Documents. U. S. Government Printing Office. Washington, D. C. 1973.

Housing for the Physically Impaired: A Guide for Planning and Design. U. S. Housing Assistance Administration. U. S. Government Printing Office. Washington, D. C. 1968.

Housing of Senior Citizens. Housing Division. Census Bureau. U. S. Department of Commerce. Superintendent of Documents. U. S. Government Printing Office. Washington, D. C. 1973.

HUD's Response to the Housing Needs of Senior Citizens. Hearing befcre Subcommittee on Housing and Consumer Interests. Select Committee on Aging. House of Representatives. Ninety-Fourth Congress. September, 1975. Superintendent of Documents. U. S. Government Printing Office. Washington, D. C. 1976.

Interfaith Conference on Housing for Senior Citizens. Proceedings. U. S. Housing and Home Finance Agency. Office of Housing for Senior Citizens. Washington, D. C. 1966.

It Can't Be Home . . . U. S. Department of Health, Education and Welfare. Public Health Service. Health Services and Mental Health Administration. National Institute of Mental Health. Publication No. (HSM) 71-9050. Superintendent of Documents. U. S. Government Printing Office. Washington, D. C. 1971.

Management of Housing for Elderly. Housing Management. U. S. Department of Housing and Urban Development. Superintendent of Documents. U. S. Government Printing Office. Washington, D. C. 1972.

Management of Public Housing for the Elderly: Training Manual. National Association of Housing and Redevelopment Officials. Washington, D. C. 1965.

Noam, Ernst. (Translated by John S. Monks). Homes for the Aged: Supervision and Standards. A Report on the Legal Situation in European Countries. Administration on Aging. U. S. Department of Health, Education and Welfare. DHEW Publication No. (OHD) 75-20104. Superintendent of Documents. U. S. Government Printing Office. Washington, D. C. 1975.

Older Americans: Facts About Incomes and Housing. U. S. Department of Housing and Urban Development. Superintendent of Documents. U. S. Government Printing Office. Washington, D. C. 1973.

Older Americans in Rural Areas. Special Committee on Aging. United States Senate. Ninety-First Congress. First Session. Superintendent of Documents. U. S. Government Printing Office. Washington, D. C. 1970.

Population, Housing and Income and Federal Housing Programs. U. S. Department of Housing and Urban Development. Superintendent of Documents. U. S. Government Printing Office. Washington, D. C. 1971.

Portraits in Community Health: The Dexter Manor Story. U. S. Department of Health, Education and Welfare. Public Health Service. Publication No. 1344-3. Superintendent of Documents. U. S. Government Printing Office. Washington, D. C. October, 1966.

Provision of Housing for Rural Elderly Under Major Federal Housing Programs. Subcommittee on Rural Development. Agriculture and Forestry Committee. United States Senate. Ninety-Third Congress. First Session. Washington, D. C. 1974.

"A Salute to the Nation's Elderly." HUD Challenge. U. S. Department of Housing and Urban Development. Washington, D. C. May, 1975.

Usefulness of the Model Cities Program to the Elderly. Hearings Before the Special Committee on Aging. United States Senate. Ninetieth Congress. Second Session. Superintendent of Documents. U. S. Government Printing Office. Washington, D. C. 1970.

MEDICARE AND MEDICAID

Feingold, Eugene. Medicare: Policy and Politics. Chandler Publishing Company. San Francisco, California. 1966.

Case study and policy analysis of medical care cost and the events leading to the health insurance law for the aged.

Greenfield, Margaret. Health Insurance for the Aged: The 1965 Program for Medicare. Institute of Governmental Studies. University of California. Berkeley, California. 1966.

Description of the 1965 Social Security Amendments and medical insurance for the aged, giving the rationale for a Federal Program; reviews the struggle for enactment.

__________. Medicare and Medicaid: The 1965 and 1967 Social Security Amendments. Institute of Governmental Studies. University of California. Berkeley, California. 1968.

Description of anticipated impact of Medicare and Medicaid provisions; useful for historical comparisons.

Marmor, Theodore R. The Politics of Medicare. Aldine Publishing Company. Chicago, Illinois. 1973.

A detailed account of the U. S. adoption of Medicare and an analysis of how the political system deals with deeply devisive social issues.

Match, Sondra K. (Editor). Health, Aging, Illness and Poverty. Senior Opportunities and Services. Technical Assistance Monograph No. 2. National Council on the Aging. Washington, D. C. 1970.

Examination of hazards of old age, sickness, and poverty, and a look at the relief afforded by Medicare and Medicaid.

Myers, Robert J. Medicare. Richard D. Irwin, Inc. Homewood, Illinois. 1970.

Legislative evolvement, program analysis, and financial experiences of Medicare and Medicaid.

Public Health and Public Responsibility: The Task Before Us. New York State Joint Legislative Committee on the Problems of Public Health and Medicare. Legislative Document No. 40. Albany, New York. 1967.

Discussion of problems in Medicaid, nursing shortages, medical costs, and conditions of municipal hospitals.

Schottland, Charles I. The Social Security Program in the United States. Second Edition. Appleton-Century-Crofts. New York, New York. 1970.

Information on Medicare, Medicaid and work incentive programs.

Schwartz, Jerome L. Medical Plans and Health Care: Consumer Participation in Policymaking, With a Special Section on Medicare. Charles C. Thomas. Springfield, Illinois. 1968.

Comparative analysis of health plans sponsored and controlled by consumers and those under control and sponsorship of physicians.

Skidmore, Max J. Medicare and the American Rhetoric of Reconciliation. University of Alabama Press. Tuscaloosa, Alabama. 1970.

An historical account of the Medicare Act; social change analysis.

Snoke, Albert W., and Somers, Anne Ramsay. Medicare and the Hospitals: Issues and Prospects. Brookings Institute. Washington, D. C. 1967.

A discussion of the impact of Medicare on various aspects of health care which includes analysis of hospital organization, financing, staffing, planning, and quality and cost control .

Somers, Herman M., and Somers, Anne R. Medicare and the Hospitals. The Brookings Institute. Washington, D. C. 1967.

Written only a few months after enactment of Medicare, this book gives the provisions of Titles XVIII and XIX of the Social Security Act. One component is the section that discusses projected trends related to Medicare and the nation's hospitals a decade ahead. This book has substantial historical value for study of this complex health insurance program.

Spiegel, Allen D., and Podair, Simon (Editors). Medicaid: Lessons for National Health Insurance. Aspen Systems Corporation. Rockville, Maryland. 1975.

A collection of thirty articles as well as overviews by the editors which relate the Medicaid experience to what the program portends for National Health Insurance.

Witkin, Erwin. The Impact of Medicare. Charles C. Thomas. Springfield, Illinois. 1971.

An historical analysis of Medicare and its impact on delivery of health care in the United States.

U. S. GOVERNMENT PUBLICATIONS

Brief Explanation of Medicare, A. Social Security Administration. DHEW Publication No. (SSA) 75-10043. U. S. Department of Health, Education and Welfare. U. S. Government Printing Office. Washington, D. C. 1975.

Corning, Peter A. The Evolution of Medicare . . . From Idea to Law. Research Report No. 29. Superintendent of Documents. U. S. Government Printing Office. Washington, D. C. 1969.

Cutbacks in Medicare and Medicaid Coverage. Subcommittee on Health of the Elderly. Special Committee on Aging. United States Senate. Ninety-second Congress. Superintendent of Documents. U. S. Government Printing Office. Washington, D. C. May 10, 1971.

Helbing, Charles. Short-Stay Hospitals Under Medicare, 1969. Office of Research and Statistics, Social Security Administration. U. S. Department of Health, Education and Welfare. DHEW Publication No. (SSA) 74-11702. Superintendent of Documents. U. S. Government Printing Office. Washington, D. C. 1973.

Improvement Needed in Administration of Program to Provide Medicare Benefits for Welfare Recipients. General Accounting Office. U. S. Department of Health, Education and Welfare. Superintendent of Documents. U. S. Government Printing Office. Washington, D. C. 1973.

Kowalczyk, George. Utilization of Short-Stay Hospitals Under Medicare by Type of Control and Bed Size. Social and Rehabilitation Service. U. S. Department of Health, Education and Welfare. Superintendent of Documents. U. S. Government Printing Office. Washington, D. C. 1973.

Medicare, 1971, Section 2: Enrollment. Office of Research and Statistics. Social Security Administration. U. S. Department of Health, Education and Welfare. DHEW Publication No. (SSA) 73-11704. Superintendent of Documents. U. S. Government Printing Office. Washington, D. C. 1973.

Medicare, Health Insurance for Aged, 1970. Office of Research and Statistics. Social Security Administration. U. S. Department of Health, Education and Welfare. DHEW Publication No. (SSA) 74-11704. Superintendent of Documents. U. S. Government Printing Office. Washington, D. C. 1973.

Medicare, Health Insurance for Aged, Amounts Reimbursed by State and County, 1971. Office of Research and Statistics. Social Security Administration. U. S. Department of Health, Education and Welfare. DHEW Publication No. (SSA) 73-11704. Superintendent of Documents. U. S. Government Printing Office. Washington, D. C. 1973.

Problems in Providing Proper Care to Medicaid and Medicare Patients in Skilled Nursing Homes. U. S. Department of Health, Education and Welfare. Report to the Congress by the Comptroller General of the United States. Superintendent of Documents. U. S. Government Printing Office. Washington, D. C. 1971.

Ruther, Martin. Medicare, General Enrollment Period for Aged, 1973. Social Security Administration. U. S. Department of Health, Education and Welfare. DHEW Publication No. (SSA) 74-11702. Superintendent of Documents. U. S. Government Printing Office. Washington, D. C. 1974.

Your Medicare Handbook. U. S. Department of Health, Education and Welfare. Social Security Administration. Superintendent of Documents. U. S. Government Printing Office. Washington, D. C. 1977. (Updated periodically)

NURSING CARE FOR THE AGED

Birchenall, Joan, and Streight, Mary Eileen. Care of the Older Adult. J. B. Lippincott Company. Philadelphia, Pennsylvania. 1973.

A discussion of the role of the nurse in preventive and restorative care. Attention is given to the aging process, associated problems and disease etiology.

Blumberg, Jeanne, E., and Drummond, Eleanor E. Nursing Care of the Long-Term Patient. Second Edition. Springer Publishing Company. New York, New York. 1971.

A model for care, and pertinent aspects of the techniques of nursing service, as well as the role of the nurse in providing emotional support to patient and family.

Brickner, Philip W. (Editor). Care of the Nursing Home Patient. The Macmillan Company. New York, New York. 1971.

Description of a total medical care program and the critical role assumed by the nursing home; includes other aspects of patient care.

Brody, Elaine M. Long-Term Care of Older People: A Practical Guide. Human Sciences Press. New York, New York. 1977.

A practical guide for workers charged with the care of those in institutions such as nursing homes and homes for the aged.

Browning, Mary H. Nursing and the Aging Patient. The American Journal of Nursing Company. New York, New York. 1974.

One volume in the Contemporary Nursing Series, it consists of a compilation of 36 articles dealing with geriatric nursing as it is practiced in a diversity of settings and geographic areas.

Buckley, Bonita Rice. Nursing Care of the aged. Revised Edition. University of Wisconsin Extension. Madison, Wisconsin. 1973.

Emphasis is upon special problems of nursing home patients.

Burnside, Irene Mortensen (Editor). Nursing and the Aged. McGraw-Hill Book Company. New York, New York. 1976.

A comprehensive treatment of broad aspects of gerontology related to nursing care of older patients.

____________________. Psychosocial Nursing Care of the Aged. McGraw-Hill Book Company. New York, New York. 1973.

Collection of papers by nurses abour relevant nursing practices in the field of psycho-social care of the aged.

Caldwell, Esther, and Hegner, Barbara R. Geriatric Nursing: A Study of Maturity. Delmar Publishers. Albany, New York. 1972.

A simply written but perceptive textbook for geriatric student nurses.

Conahan, Judith M. Helping Your Elderly Patients: A Guide for Nursing Assistants. The Tiresias Press. New York, New York. 1976.

Emphasis is upon psychosocial care of the institutionalized aged.

Falconer, Mary, et al. Aging Patients: A Guide to Their Care. Springer Publishing Company. New York, New York. 1976.

Title self explanatory.

Gunter, Laurie M., and Ryan, Joanne E. Self-Assessment of Current Knowledge in Geriatric Nursing. Medical Examination Publishing Company. Flushing, New York. 1976.

A continuing education resource, covering basic knowledge, nursing concepts, clinical aspects, nutrition and other topics.

Hodkinson, Mary A. Nursing the Elderly. Pergamon Publishing Company. New York, New York. 1966.

A general discussion of procedures and problems in nursing the aged with attention to the care of patients with specific disorders.

Hooper, Langdon, and McWilliams, Paul A.(Editors). _Care of the Nursing Home Patient_. Little, Brown and Company. Boston, Massachusetts. 1967.

A comprehensive discussion of numerous aspects of care for the aged patient. Offers information necessary for quality patient care applicable to nurse aides, nursing assistants, orderlies, and attendants in nursing homes and other extended care institutions.

How to Be A Nurse's Aide in a Nursing Home. American Health Care Association. Washington, D. C. 1975.

A handbook for the nursing aide. Designed as a self-teaching guide or as a supplement of in-service training.

Moe, Mildred I. _For Patient's Sake: A Book for All Personnel Who Care for the Aged_. Geriatric Care. Minneapolis, Minnesota. 1972.

Based upon the long clinical nursing experience of the author, the book discusses aspects of nursing service in nursing homes and related care facilities. Subjects include: quality of nursing care, philosophy of geriatric nursing, nurse-patient relations, physician-nurse relations, etc.

Monea, Helen Elena. _Instructor's Manual: Nursing and the Aged_. McGraw-Hill Company. New York, New York. 1976.

A helpful tool for the instructor, especially for a field instructor working with students assigned to a long-term care facility for the elderly. Includes lesson plans correlated with experential learning.

Newton, Kathleen. _Geriatric Nursing_. C. V. Mosby Company. St. Louis, Missouri. 1966.

A broad background of problems of aging and a discussion of preventive care measures.

Nursing Digest Focus on Care of the Elderly. Prepared by the "Nursing Digest," Editorial Staff. Contemporary Publishing, Inc. Wakefield, Massachusetts. 1975.

Coverage includes varied aspects of care and maintenance for the aged.

O'Brien, Maureen J. The Care of the Elderly Person: A Guide for the Licensed Practical Nurse. The C. V. Mosby Company. St. Louis, Missouri. 1975.

Textbook designed for student practical nurses and licensed practical nurses; approaches nursing care by emphasis upon comprehension of the dynamics of aging.

O'Carm, Sister Joseph Mary. Complete Manual of Geriatric Nursing. Impress House. New York, New York. 1973.

Subjects include disease etiology and nursing procedures. A good bibliography is provided for further study.

Rudd, Thomas Newton. The Nursing of the Elderly Sick: A Practical Handbook of Geriatric Nursing. Faber and Faber. London, England. 1970.

Practical application of nursing knowledge and procedures to problems confronting personnel involved in the care of geriatric patients.

Stevens, C. B. Special Needs of Long-Term Patients. J. B. Lippincott Company. Philadelphia, Pennsylvania. 1974.

Consideration is given to specialized aspects of nursing care during prolonged illness, and to the fact that many long-term patients are elderly.

Stevens, Marion K. Geriatric Nursing for Practical Nurses. Second Edition. W. B. Saunders Company. Philadelphia, Pennsylvania. 1975.

An introduction to the special needs and difficulties of the older patient, identifies ways in which this patient differs from younger, medical-surgical patients.

Stolten, Jane H. The Geriatric Aide. Little, Brown and Company. Boston, Massachusetts. 1973.

A practical help for nurse trainees, nurse practitioners, and geriatric aides which provides a basis for understanding the emotional and physical needs of older patients and how to meet these needs.

Storrs, Alison. Geriatric Nursing. (Nurse's Aide Series) Williams and Wilkins Company. Baltimore, Maryland. 1976.

A book written primarily for student nurses interested in geriatrics, it has value for graduate nurses as well. Since the author is British, she reflects the view of geriatrics as a professional and a paraprofessional specialty. Included are: the geriatric care unit, disorders prevalent and an appendix on equipment for a geriatric unit.

Weiss, James. Nurses, Patients and Social Systems. University of Missouri Press. Columbia, Missouri. 1968.

Emphasis focuses upon the effects of skilled nursing intervention upon institutionalized older adults.

U. S. GOVERNMENT PUBLICATIONS

Elementary Rehabilitation Nursing Care. Public Health Service, Division of Nursing. Publication No. 1436. U. S. Department of Health, Education and Welfare. U. S. Government Printing Office. Washington, D. C. 1966.

Portraits in Community Health: Rural Home Nursing Care for Long-Term Illness. U. D. Department of Health, Education and Welfare. Public Health Service. Publication No. 1344-1. Superintendent of Documents. U. S. Government Printing Office. Washington, D. C. 1965.

NURSING HOMES

Accreditation Manual for Long Term Care Facilities. Second Edition. Joint Commission on Accreditation of Hospitals. 975 North Michigan Avenue, Chicago, Illinois 60611. 1975.

The revised standards and criteria for accreditation of long term care facilities. These standards constitute a floor of minimum provisions and services.

Anson, Robert E., Jr. Nursing Home Ombudsman Training Manual. (Revised) Citizens for Better Care. 960 East Jefferson Avenue. Detroit, Michigan 48207. 1976.

A resource manual which identifies common problem areas in long-term care facilities, problem analysis, consequences, and prevention and solution approaches.

____________________ (Editor). Organizer's Manual for Nursing Home Ombudsmen. Citizens for Better Care. 960 East Jefferson Avenue. Detroit, Michigan 48207. 1976.

A handbook to assist ombudsmen programs and other advocacy groups in program organization, development and training.

Braverman, Jordan. Nursing Home Standards: A Tragic Dilemma in American Health. American Pharmaceutical Association. Washington, D. C. 1970.

An examination of administration, patient care, environmental health, fire and safety standards for nursing homes not only nationally, but also by state and region.

Burk, Doris M. The Forgotten Family Jewels. Vantage Books. New York, New York. 1974.

A book which over glorifies nursing homes in the U. S., perpetuates myths which professionals are working to destroy, and takes positions which research does not support.

Buttaro, Peter J. Legal Manual for Nursing Homes. Western Printing Company. Aberdeen, South Dakota. 1972.

Text written by an attorney; considers the legal aspects of nursing home administration, including corporate negligence, liability, licensure and labor laws.

Desnick, Shirley G. *Geriatric Contentment: A Guide to its Achievement in Your Home*. Charles C. Thomas. Springfield, Illinois. 1971.

This book deals with life in a nursing home, emphasizing patient individuality; gives attention also to recreational programs.

Douglas, Ellen. *Apostles of Light*. Houghton-Mifflin Company. Boston, Massachusetts. 1973.

A novel concerned with negative aspects of being old in American society. The story incorporates a plea for realization of the effects of indifference and sometimes inhumane treatment of the elderly by relatives and by personnel in nursing homes.

Eastman, C. Alexander. *The Sin of Caring*. Metropolitan Press. Portland, Oregon. 1974.

The case history of a nursing home in North Idaho which was forced to close as the result of Federal regulations.

Faunce, Frances Avery. *The Nursing Home Visitor: A Handbook Written from the Inside*. Abingdon Press. Nashville, Tennessee. 1969.

A guide emphasizing the need for visitors to understand the viewpoint of the patient. Gives specific suggestions.

Fire Safety Manual for Nursing Homes. American Nursing Home Association. Washington, D. C. (N.D.)

A guide to fire safety in the nursing home environment.

Fire Test in a Nursing Home Patient Room. American Health Care Association. Washington, D. C. 1975.

A report of the result and recoomendations from the AHCA fire safety program tests; covers such areas as automatic sprinklers, smoke detectors, life safety criteria, interior finish, doors.

Garvin, Richard M., and Burger, Robert E. *Where They Go to Die: The Tragedy of America's Aged*. Delacorte Press. New York, New York. 1968.

Detailed consideration of convalescent facilities, nursing homes, rest homes and homes for the aged which can serve as a guide in selecting suitable living arrangements; includes what to seek and what to avoid.

Gottesman, Leonard E. (Editor). "Symposium - Long-Term Care: Research, Policy and Practice." The Gerontologist. Vol. 14. December, 1974.

This issue includes six papers on research relevant to nursing homes. Topics cover: relocation and social policy, alternatives in life patterns, accountability, variances in facilities, and quality of care.

Gubrium, Jaber F. Living and Dying at Murray Manor. St. Martin's Press. New York, New York. 1975.

A detailed descriptive analysis of life in a nursing home-home for the aged, which describes the activities and social organization of top staff, floor staff, patients and residents.

Henry, Jules. Culture Against Man. Vintage Books. New York, New York. 1965.

Part Three, Chapter 10, "Human Obsolescence," contains worthwhile comments on nursing homes and nursing care for the aged.

How to Choose a Nursing Home. Institute of Gerontology. University of Michigan. Ann Arbor, Michigan. 1974.

A guide published jointly with Citizens for Better Care to be used in selecting a nursing home, with suggestions for alternatives to institutional care. Printed in large type for use by older persons.

Jones, Donald D., and Follman, J. F., Jr. Health Insurance and Nursing Home Care: A Study. Health Insurance Association of America. Chicago, Illinois. 1969.

Descriptive analysis of nursing home care in the United States, its costs, utilization, and coverage by private health insurance.

Kinney, Mark B. Staff Development in Geriatric Institutions. Institute of Gerontology. University of Michigan. Ann Arbor, Michigan. 1976.

Title self explanatory.

Koncelik, Joseph A. *Designing the Open Nursing Home*. Dowden, Hutchinson & Ross. Stroudsburg, Pennsylvania. 1976.

A resource book based upon research on physical, social and psychological characteristics of the infirm aged: includes recommendations about architectural and interior design, furnishings and other equipment.

__________________, et al. *The New Nursing Home: Conference Proceedings*. College of Human Ecology. Cornell University. Ithaca, New York. 1973.

Consideration is given to the nursing home role and responsibilities.

Kramer, Charles H., and Kramer, Jeannette R. *Basic Principles of Long-Term Patient Care*. Charles C. Thomas. Springfield, Illinois. 1976.

Drawing upon personal experience in nursing home administration, the complexity of therapeutic geriatric care is discussed. Another section covers the establishment of a program of total therapeutic care.

Long Term Care in Perspective: Past, Present and Future Directions. American Nurses' Association. Kansas City, Missouri. 1975.

A collection of papers presented in the meeting of the American Academy of Nursing which covers topics such as, status of care, evaluation, economics and politics of care.

Markus, Elliot J. *Post-Relocation Mortality Among Institutionalized Aged: A Report on Two Studies Conducted by the Benjamin Rose Institute*. Benjamin Rose Institute. Cleveland, Ohio. 1970.

Report on an investigation of the elderly person's reactions to moving from private dwellings to institutional facilities.

McGlaun, Mabel D. *A Handbook for Recreation in the Modern Nursing Home*. B-Mac Publications. Garland, Texas. 1972.

Guidelines for recreation programs in nursing homes written by a former recreation director for Manor Homes of Dallas.

Mendelson, Mary Adelaide. Tender Loving Greed. Alfred A. Knopf. New York, New York. 1974.

An impressionistic book devoted to a scathing attack on the business aspects of nursing homes in the United States. The stated purpose is to show the public and the medical profession the realities of aging and the poor care often provided to older persons.

Moos, Rudolph H. Evaluating Treatment Environments. John Wiley and Sons. New York, New York. 1974.

The author approaches the environment of the facility in which treatment is given from the standpoint of its sociological impact.

Moreland Act Commission Reports. Office of the New York State Moreland Act Commission. New York State Legislature. Albany, New York.

1. Regulating Nursing Home Care: The Paper Tigers, 1975.

   This report deals with setting and enforcing standards of care in nursing homes and other health related facilities.

2. Reimbursement of Nursing Home Property Costs: Pruning the Money Tree, 1976.

   The second report deals with the real estate aspects of nursing home and residential facilities operations. A new system is offered for reimbursement of property costs of proprietary homes.

3. Political Influence and Political Accountability: One Foot In the Door, 1976.

   A description of the political system under which Medicaid fraud and patient abuse occurred among some of the New York City nursing homes.

4. Nursing Homes and Domiciliary Facility Planning: Decisions on the Back of An Envelope, 1976.

   The subject in this report is new construction of long term care facilities, planning procedures, and methods for certifying need. Questions are raised in all of the above areas, and reasons given for halting construction.

5. Reimbursing Operating Cost: Dollars Without Sense, 1976.

The fifth report reviews Federal reimbursement programs for operating costs in nursing homes, other health related and domiciliary care facilities, as well as the New York State Department of Health System. Problems are identified and recommendations made.

6. Assessment and Placement: Anything Goes, 1976.

An exposition of inadequate assessment of needs, placements unrelated to specific needs, biases affecting decision and lack of standards and controls. Reforms are proposed.

7. Long Term Care Regulation: Past Lapses, Future Prospects, 1976.

This report summarizes the findings by the Commission and the previous reports. It deals with the need to measure quality of care and regulatory controls as well as the need for an advocate for the aging. Legislative proposals are made.

Nassau, Jean B. Choosing a Nursing Home. Funk and Wagnalls. New York, New York. 1975.

A guide for locating a nursing home that offers quality care and for understanding the types and quality of professional care to which the patient is legally entitled.

Nursing Home Fact Book. The American Nursing Home Association. Washington, D. C. (Updated periodically.)

Information on development, trends and problems in the nursing home industry.

Rabinowitz, Dorothy, and Nielson, Yedida. Home Life. The Macmillan Company. New York, New York. 1971.

A description of what can occur in a nursing home which is not committed to the best interest of the patients.

Rooke, M. Leigh, and Wingrove, C. Ray. Long Term Care Facilities Management: An Annotated Bibliography. Virginia Commonwealth University. Richmond, Virginia. 1974.

Title self explanatory.

Routh, Thomas A. Choosing a Nursing Home: The Problems and Their Solutions. Charles C. Thomas. Springfield, Illinois. 1970.

Practical information for use by those who work with the aged, and who seek a better understanding of the elderly and their problems.

______________. Nursing Homes: A Blessing or a Curse. Charles C. Thomas. Springfield, Illinois. 1968.

A collection of previously published articles concerned with social work related to nursing homes.

Sarton, Mary. As We Are Now. W. W. Norton. New York, New York. 1973.

A novel that focuses on one old woman who is trying to survive in a nursing home located in a remote rural area. Constitutes an indictment of sentencing elderly persons to unpleasantness in their late years.

Summary of States' Licensure Requirements for Nursing Home Administrators. Compiled by the Department of Education, Research and Development. American College of Nursing Home Administrators. Silver Spring, Maryland. 1975.

Title self explanatory.

Thomas, William C., Jr. Nursing Homes and Public Policy: Drift and Decision in New York State. Cornell University Press. Ithaca, New York. 1969.

A survey of public policy for nursing homes in New York State; examines the effect of Federal, State, and local laws on institutions caring for the ill aged.

Tobin, Sheldon S., and Lieberman, Morton A. Last Home for the Aged. Jossey-Bass Publishers. San Francisco, California. 1976.

A study of the critical implications of institutionalization which finds that more extensive psychological damage may occur prior to the actual institutionalization.

Townsend, Claire. Old Age: The Last Segregation. Grossman Publishers. New York, New York. 1971.

Ralph Nader Study Group Report on Nursing Homes is based upon official interviews, reports, correspondence, as well as observations and interviews in nursing homes. Includes recommendations and references.

Tulloch, G. Janet. A Home is Not a Home: Life Within a Nursing Home. Seabury Press. New York, New York. 1976.

A fictional account of life in a nursing home written by a resident. The foreword is written by Senator Charles Percy.

U. S. GOVERNMENT PUBLICATIONS

Assessing Health Care Needs in Skilled Nursing Facilities: Health Professional Perspectives. Long Term Care Facility Improvement Campaign. Monograph No. 1. U. S. Department of Health, Education and Welfare. Public Health Service, Office of Nursing Home Affairs. DHEW Publication No. (OS) 77-50049. Washington, D. C. 1976.

Directory of Nursing Home Facilities. (4 Volumes). U. S. Department of Health, Education and Welfare. National Center for Health Statistics. NCHS,Office of Scientific and Technical Information. Superintendent of Documents. U. S. Government Printing Office. Washington, D. C.

Northeast Volume - 1975.
North Central Volume - 1975.
South Volume - 1975.
Western Volume - (in press).

Errors in Fire Safety Inspections of Nursing Homes. Hearing Before a Subcommittee on Government Operations. House of Representatives. Ninety-Third Congress. Second Session. Superintendent of Documents. U. S. Government Printing Office. Washington, D. C. 1974.

Fire Safety Deficiencies in Nursing Homes. Twenty-Fourth Report by the Committee on Government Operations. Ninety-Third Congress. Second Session. House Report No. 93-1627. Superintendent of Documents. U. S. Government Printing Office. Washington, D. C. December, 1974.

Guide for Social Services in Nursing Homes and Related Facilities, A. U. S. Department of Health, Education and Welfare. Public Health Service. Publication No. 1878. Superintendent of Documents. U. S. Government Printing Office. Washington, D. C. Reprinted 1969.

Long-Term Care Facility Improvement Study, Introductory Report. Office of Nursing Home Affairs. Public Health Service. U. S. Department of Health, Education and Welfare. Washington, D. C. 1975.

McKnight, Eleanor M. *Nursing Home Research Study: Quantitative Measurement of Nursing Services.* U. S. Department of Health, Education and Welfare. Public Health Service. National Institutes of Health. Bureau of Health Manpower Education. Division of Nursing. Superintendent of Documents. U. S. Government Printing Office. Washington, D. C. 1971.

Mental Health: Principles and Training Techniques in Nursing Home Care. National Institute of Mental Health. Rockville, Maryland. 1972.

Noncompletion of Nursing Home Fire Safety Plans. Hearing Before a Subcommittee of the Committee on Government Operations. House of Representatives. Ninety-Third Congress. Second Session. Superintendent of Documents. U. S. Government Printing Office. Washington, D. C. August, 1974.

Nursing Home Care in the United States: Failure in Public Policy. Introductory Report of the Subcommittee on Long Term Care, Special Committee on Aging. United States Senate. Superintendent of Documents. U. S. Government Printing Office. Washington, D. C. 1974-1976.

Nursing Homes, A County and Metropolitan Area Data Book. Department of Health, Education and Welfare. Superintendent of Documents. U. S. Government Printing Office. Washington, D. C. 1974.

Nursing Homes and Related Health Care Facilities. U. S. Training and Employment Service. Industry Manpower Surveys. No. 116. Superintendent of Documents. U. S. Government Printing Office. Washington, D. C. 1969.

Selected Characteristics of Nursing Homes for Aged and Chronically Ill, United States, June-August, 1969. Division of Health Resources Statistics. National Center for Health Statistics. U. S. Department of Health, Education and Welfare. DHEW Publication No. (HRA) 74-1513. Superintendent of Documents. U. S. Government Printing Office. Washington, D. C. 1974.

Selected Operating and Financial Characteristics of Nursing Homes, United States, 1973-74 National Nursing Home Survey. Superintendent of Documents. U. S. Government Printing Office. Washington, D. C. 1975.

Survey of FHA-Assisted Nursing Homes. U. S. Department of Housing and Urban Development. Superintendent of Documents. U. S. Government Printing Office. Washington, D. C. 1969.

Trends in Long-Term Care. Hearing Before the Special Committee on Aging. United States Senate. Ninety-Fourth Congress. First Session. February 19, 1975. Superintendent of Documents. U. S. Government Printing Office. Washington, D. C. 1976.

Trends in Long-Term Care. Hearings Before Special Committee on Aging. Subcommittee on Long-Term Care, Parts 1-25. United States Senate. Superintendent of Documents. U. S. Government Printing Office. Washington, D. C. 1972-1975.

What Can Be Done in Nursing Homes, Positive Aspects in Long-Term Care. Subcommittee on Long-Term Care, Special Committee on Aging. United States Senate. Ninety-Fourth Congress. First Session. Superintendent of Documents. U. S. Government Printing Office. Washington, D. C. 1975.

NUTRITION AND FOOD

Ahrens, Richard A. Nutrition for Health. Wadsworth Publishing Company, Inc. Belmont, California. 1970.

Emphasis is upon the need to consider the critical importance of nutrition in relation to health.

Bogert, Lydia Jean, et al. Nutrition and Physical Fitness. W. B. Saunders Company. Philadelphia, Pennsylvania. 1973.

Chapter 23 deals with nutrition for older people.

Braver, Ruth C. Chicago Nutrition Program for Older Adults. Mayor's Office for Senior Citizens. Chicago, Illinois. 1972.

Report on a study of a three-year nutrition program in Chicago.

Exton-Smith, A. N., and Scott, D. L. (Editors). Vitamins in the Elderly. Report of the Proceedings of a Symposium held at the Royal College of Physicians. London England. May 2, 1968. J. Wright Publishers. Bristol, England. 1968.

Discussion of adequate nutrition for the aged and the consequences of inadequacy.

Golden Spoon: Recipes for One or Two, The. Senior Citizens Centers of Greater Minneapolis. 1627 South Sixth Street. Minneapolis, Minnesota 55454.

A cookbook in large type which emphasizes low cost and high nutrition; includes low sodium and sugar free diets.

Hamilton, Donna M. The After-50 Cookbook. Swallow Press. Chicago, Illinois. 1974.

A cookbook that seeks to offer a creative approach to cooking for one or two persons, with an emphasis upon retired person needs and those on special diets.

Holmes, Douglas, and Howell, Sandra. Guidelines for Nutrition Programs. Center for Community Research. 33 West 60th Street. New York, New York. 1972.

Title self explanatory.

Home-Delivered Meals for the Ill, Handicapped and Elderly. National Council on the Aging. Washington, D. C. 1965.

Guidelines for the establishment, operation and financing of programs for home-delivered meals, with particular attention to the quality of service. Includes a descriptive analysis of five types of programs.

Howell, Sandra C., and Loeb, Martin B. "Nutrition and Aging: A Monograph for Practitioners." The Gerontologist. Vol. 9, No. 3. Autumn, 1969.

This monograph is divided into two sections - Nutrition, Health and Society: Research Review; and Nutrition Programming for the Older Adult: Patterns, Problems, and Processes.

Johnson, Harry J. Eat, Drink, Be Merry, and Live Longer. Doubleday and Company, Inc. New York, New York. 1968.

Emphasis is on the role of good nutrition during middle age for prolonged health maintenance.

Kahrl, William L. Food Service on a Budget: For Schools, Senior Citizens, Colleges, Nursing Homes, Hospitals, Industrial and Correctional Institutions. Cahners Books. Boston, Massachusetts. 1974.

A book designed to aid operators of food service facilities concerned with feeding large numbers of people. Deals with planning, operation, design, layout and remodeling.

Kinderlehrer, Jane. How to Feel Younger Longer. Rodale Press. Emmaus, Pennsylvania. 1976.

A very readable book on nutrition written by the Senior Editor of Prevention Magazine.

Klinger, Judith L., et al (Editors). Mealtime Manual for the Aged and Handicapped. Institute of Rehabilitative Medicine. New York University Medical Center. Simon & Schuster, Inc. New York, New York. 1970.

A demonstration of how kitchen tasks can be streamlined to permit the aged and disabled to live active lives. Includes information on nutrition and foods that can be prepared simply.

Krause, Marie V., and Hunscher, Martha A. Food, Nutrition and Diet Therapy. W. B. Saunders Company. Philadelphia, Pennsylvania. 1972.

Chapter 15 deals with geriatric nutrition.

Mass Media and Nutrition Education. Society for Nutrition Education. 2140 Shattuck Avenue, Suite 1110. Bevereley, California 94704.

A compilation of readings from the Journal of Education and the Society for Nutrition Education Newsletter which includes such topics as the role of mass media in nutrition education, planning and implementing mass media nutrition education programs, reaching and influencing mass media, and regulations affecting food advertising.

Meals on Wheels Manual. Lutheran Service Society of Western Pennsylvania. Pittsburgh, Pennsylvania. 1973.

A description of how to set up and operate a Meals-on-Wheels program.

Minocha, S. L. Nutrition and Our Over-Populated Planet. Charles C. Thomas. Springfield, Illinois. 1975.

This book includes a chapter on nutritional needs in old age.

National Diet-Heart Study: Final Report, The. Monograph No. 18. American Heart Association. New York, New York. 1968.

Recommendations from large scale studies on the prevention of coronary heart disease in middle-aged men using dietary procedures.

Nutrition and Nutrition Programs for Older People. National Council on the Aging. Washington, D. C. (Revised periodically.)

An annotated bibliography.

Nutrition and Social Interaction Among the Aged: Pilot Study 1968-1970. Final Report. Oklahoma University. Tulsa, Oklahoma. 1970.

A description of Tulsa's model cities' nutrition and dining project.

Rockstein, Morris, and Sussman, Marvin L. (Editors). Nutrition, Longevity, and Aging. Academic Press. New York, New York. 1976.

Topics covered include biochemical effects of nutrition, protein metabolism, vitamins, nutritional aspects in care of persons with special diseases, and others.

Wagner, Willett Gertrude. Group Meals for Senior Citizens in a Community Setting: A Procedural Manual. The Hudson Guild Senior Association. New York, New York. 1972.

A monograph which offers a plan for serving nutritious main meals to persons 60 years of age and over, five times a week.

Welfare Planning Council of Dade County. Evaluation of Low Cost Meals Programs. Senior Citizens of Dade County. Miami, Florida. 1968.

An evaluation study report of the Dade County, Florida, Senior Center low cost lunch program.

Winick, Myron (Editor). Nutrition and Development. John Wiley and Sons, Inc. New York, New York. 1972.

A technical book synthesizing existing knowledge about nutrition and human development. Evidence shows that nutrition during early life can have a lasting influence on development of the organism into later life.

U. S. GOVERNMENT PUBLICATIONS

Bechill, William D., and Wolgamot, Irene. Nutrition for the Elderly. Administration on Aging. U. S. Department of Health, Education and Welfare. DHEW Publication No. (SRS) 72-20236. Superintendent of Documents. U. S. Government Printing Office. Washington, D.C. 1973.

Coble, M. Catherine. Guide to Nutrition and Food Service for Nursing Homes and Homes for the Aged. Community Health Service. U. S. Department of Health, Education and Welfare. DHEW Publication No. (HSM) 71-6701. Superintendent of Documents. U. S. Government Printing Office. Washington, D. C. Revised 1972.

Elderly Americans' Nutritional Needs. Select Committee on Nutrition and Human Needs. Ninety-third Congress. First Session. U. S. Senate. Superintendent of Documents. U. S. Government Printing Office. Washington, D. C. 1974.

Guide to Nutrition and Food Service for Nursing Homes and Homes for Aged, A. U. S. Department of Health, Education and Welfare. Public Health Service. Publication No. 1309. Superintendent of Documents. U. S. Government Printing Office. Washington, D. C. Revised 1971.

Guidelines for Dietitians and Public Health Nutritionists in Home Health Services. U. S. Department of Health, Education and Welfare. Public Health Service. Publication No. 1794. Health Services and Mental Health Administration. Community Health Service. Superintendent of Documents. U. S. Government Printing Office. Washington, D. C. Revised 1970.

Home Delivered Meals: A National Directory. U. S. Administration on Aging. Superintendent of Documents. U. S. Government Printing Office. Washington, D. C. 1971.

Nutrition for the Elderly: The AOA Experience - Developmental Projects. U. S. Department of Health, Education and Welfare. Social and Rehabilitation Service. Administration on Aging. Washington, D. C. 1972.

Nutrition Program for the Elderly Under Older Americans Act of 1965. Ninety-second Congress. U. S. Senate. Superintendent of Documents. U. S. Government Printing Office. Washington, D. C. 1972.

Older Americans Nutrition Program. Select Subcommittee on Education. Education and Labor Committee. Ninety-third Congress. Second Session. U. S. House of Representatives. Superintendent of Documents. U. S. Government Printing Office. Washington, D. C. 1974.

Page, Louise, et al. Nutrition Program for the Elderly: A Guide to Menu Planning, Buying, and the Care of Food for Community Programs. U. S. Department of Agriculture. Agricultural Research Service. Consumer and Food Economics Institute. Washington, D. C. 1975.

Pelcovits, Jeannette, and Holmes, Douglas. Nutrition for Older Americans: Demonstration Program Experience. U. S. Department of Health, Education and Welfare. Social and Rehabilitation Service. Administration on Aging. Superintendent of Documents. U. S. Government Printing Office. Washington, D. C. 1970.

Research in Aging and Nutrition Programs for the Elderly, 1971. Subcommittee on Aging. Ninety-second Congress. First Session. Superintendent of Documents. U. S. Government Printing Office. Washington, D. C. 1971.

Simko, Margaret D., and Colitz, Karen. Nutrition and Aging: Selected Annotated Bibliography, 1964-1972. Administration on Aging. U. S. Department of Health, Education and Welfare. DHEW Publication No. (SRS) 73-20237. Superintendent of Documents. U. S. Government Printing Office. Washington, D. C. 1973.

Todhunter, E. Neige. Nutrition: Background Paper. White House Conference on Aging, 1971. National Planning Board. Background and Issues. Volume 7. Superintendent of Documents. U. S. Government Printing Office. Washington, D. C. 1971.

Walker, Mabel A., and Hill, Mary M. Food Guide for Older Folks. Consumer and Food Economics Research Division. Agricultural Research Service. U. S. Department of Agriculture. Superintendent of Documents. U. S. Government Printing Office. Washington, D. C. Revised 1972.

White House Conference on Food, Nutrition and Health: Final Report. Superintendent of Documents. U. S. Government Printing Office. Washington, D. C. 1970.

PROTECTIVE AND LEGAL SERVICES

Advocate's Handbook, The National Senior Citizens Law Center. California Rural Legal Assistance Office. San Francisco, California. 1972.

An aid to workers with the elderly in assisting them to secure legal and other benefits for which they are eligible. Emphasis is upon the advocacy role.

Alexander, George J., and Lewin, Travis H. D. The Aged and the Need for Surrogate Management. Syracuse University Press. Syracuse, New York. 1973.

Two law professors have researched surrogate management laws in the United States, and concluded that they work to the disadvantage of those they are purported to protect. A valuable resource not only to researchers, but also to those concerned with the welfare and needs of older citizens.

Blenkner, Margaret, et al. Final Report, Protective Services for Older People: Findings from the Benjamin Rose Institute Study. The Benjamin Rose Institute. Cleveland, Ohio. 1974.

Description of a controlled demonstration project to test the effectiveness of a program of protective services which represented the "best" social work thinking and practice. Results were not those expected, since the control group fared better than the experimental. The authors concluded that "intensive service of the sort supplied in the project with heavy reliance on custodial care may actually accelerate decline."

Crucial Issue in Social Work Practice: Protective Services for Older People, A. National Conference on Social Welfare. National Council on the Aging. Washington, D. C. 1966.

Discussion of protective services for the aged by experts in the legal, medical, and social work professions.

Hall, Gertrude, H., and Mathiasen, Geneva (Editors). Guide to Development of Protective Services for Older People. Charles C. Thomas. Springfield, Illinois. 1973.

Report of a study based on three community demonstration programs sponsored by the National Council on the Aging and the National Institute of Mental Health. Guidelines are derived from this experience.

Hall, Gertrude H., and Mathiasen, Geneva. Overcoming Barriers to Protective Services for the Aged. National Council on the Aging, Inc. Washington, D. C. 1968.

Offers a framework for action in establishing services to protect the impaired aged.

Heyman, Dorothy (Editor). Legal Problems of the Elderly. Center for the Study of Aging and Human Development. Duke University Medical Center. Durham, North Carolina. 1975.

Papers presented at a symposium co-sponsored by the Duke University Center for the Study of Aging and the School of Law. Topics addressed included supplemental security income, Social Security benefits, pensions, services delivery, among others.

Law and Aging Manual, The. Legal Research and Services for the Elderly. National Council of Senior Citizens, Inc. Washington, D. C. 1976.

The report of a study of legal problems facing aged persons and of services both needed and available. Offers guidance for developing legal resources for older persons at state and community levels.

Law and the Impaired Older Person: Protection or Punishment, The. The National Council on the Aging. Washington, D. C. 1966.

A monograph presenting a case study that describes the plight of an elderly woman involuntarily committed to a mental hospital. Review of the case by an attorney, a psychiatrist, and other professionals is reported. Emphasis is upon legal protective services and assignment of responsibility.

Legislative Approaches to the Problems of the Elderly: A Handbook of Model State Statutes. Legal Research and Services for the Elderly. National Council of Senior Citizens. Washington, D. C. 1971.

A comprehensive review of state statutes affecting the elderly and recommendations for a cohesive uniform legislative plan by states. Includes model laws.

Lewis, James A. (Editor). Law and Aging. School of Law. Duke University. Durham, North Carolina. 1975.

Report of the proceedings of a conference to examine laws and programs related to the elderly. Topics include Social Security, Supplemental Security Income (S.S.I.), Medicare and Medicaid, Social Services Amendments of 1974 (Title XX), the Older Americans Act, Commitment, and Protective Services. Although there is a strong emphasis upon North Carolina State statutes in several areas, contents have much wider applicability.

Protective and Legal Services for the Elderly. National Council on the Aging. Washington, D. C. (Revised periodically.)

An annotated bibliography.

Terris, Bruce J. Legal Services for the Elderly. Senior Opportunities and Services. Technical Assistance Monograph No. 9. National Council on the Aging. Washington, D. C. February, 1972.

A report on the projects designed to provide legal services to the elderly. Since not all projects were successful, this report gives experience from which other communities can plan their own programs.

Wasser, Edna. Protective Casework Practice With Older People: An Explication of the Service Component in the Benjamin Rose Institute. The Benjamin Rose Institute. Cleveland, Ohio. 1974.

Based upon a 1967 agency report and casebook, this book is concerned with the essentials of direct service to mentally impaired, non-institutionalized old people.

U. S. GOVERNMENT PUBLICATIONS

Allen, Richard D. Legal Rights of the Disabled and Disadvantaged. U. S. Department of Health, Education and Welfare. SRS-117. Superintendent of Documents. U. S. Government Printing Office. Washington, D. C. 1969.

Horowitz, Gideon, and Estes, Carol. Protective Services for the Aged. Administration on Aging. U. S. Department of Health, Education and Welfare. Superintendent of Documents. U. S. Government Printing Office. Washington, D. C. 1971.

Improving Legal Representation for Older Americans. Joint Hearing Before the Special Committee on Aging and the Subcommittee on Representation of Citizen Interests of the Committee on the Judiciary. United States Senate. Superintendent of Documents. U. S. Government Printing Office. Washington, D. C. 1974.

Legal Problems Affecting Older Americans. Special Committee on Aging. United States Senate. Ninety-first Congress. Second Session. Superintendent of Documents. U. S. Government Printing Office. Washington, D. C. 1971.

Protection for the Elderly. Consumer Bulletin No. 9. Federal Trade Commission. Superintendent of Documents. U. S. Government Printing Office. Washington, D. C. 1971.

Protective and Social Support. White House Conference on Aging. Superintendent of Documents. U. S. Government Printing Office. Washington, D. C. 1972.

Report of National Protective Services Project for Older Adults. Community Services Administration. U. S. Department of Health, Education and Welfare. DHEW Publication No. (SRS) 72-23008. Superintendent of Documents. U. S. Government Printing Office. Washington, D. C. 1971.

You, The Law, and Retirement. Administration on Aging. AOA Publication No. 800. Superintendent of Documents. U. S. Government Printing Office. Washington, D. C. 1965.

RECREATION AND LEISURE

Boyack, Virginia L. Time on Our Hands: The Problem of Leisure. Ethel Percy Andrus Gerontology Center. University of Southern California. Los Angeles, California. 1973.

Suggestions and guidelines for more effective use of leisure.

Cross, Gertrude (Editor). Senior Citizens Travel Manual. Flint Recreation and Park Board. Flint, Michigan. 1969.

A monograph giving guidelines for group travel for older persons and a model for organization of the group.

Education Program Ideas: Recreation for the Elderly, Innovations Today: Programs Tomorrow. Bureau of Continuing Education. State University of New York. Albany, New York. 1968.

A manual describing illustrative workable programs, and the administrative and program methods to be used.

Fish, Harriet U. Activities Programs for Senior Citizens. Parker Publishing Company. West Nyack, New York. 1971.

Guidelines for establishing and administering activities programs in care facilities and centers for the aged.

Gould, Elaine, and Gould, Loren. Crafts for the Elderly. Charles C. Thomas. Springfield, Illinois. 1971.

Description of 75 tested craft activities especially designed or modified to meet the needs of the aged in nursing homes.

Incani, Albert G., et al. Coordinated Activity Programs for the Aged: A How-To-Do-It Manual. American Hospital Association. Chicago, Illinois. 1975.

Guidelines for developing and directing an activity department in a long-term health care institution; gives detailed instructions for a number of activities.

Kaminsky, Marc. What's Inside You - It Shines Out of You. Horizon Press. New York, New York. 1974.

The author discusses his work with elderly persons and the therapeutic use of poetry in a recreational program.

Kleemeier, Robert W. (Editor). _Aging and Leisure: A Research Perspective into the Meaningful Use of Time_. Oxford University Press. New York, New York. 1961.

Although an old resource, this volume includes worthwhile discussions of retirement, meaning of time, and use of leisure. Some selections are specific and based on empirical research while others are general and theoretical.

Kubie, Susan H., and Landau, Gertrude. _Group Work With the Aged_. International Universities Press, Inc. New York, New York. 1969.

The authors describe nine years of work in a recreation center for the aged; written in the hope that much trial and error can be eliminated from similar programs in the future.

Leap: _Program Recreational Activities for Peppy Older People_. Aging and Aged Project. Phoenix, Arizona. 1970.

Description of a variety of programs and recreational activities used successfully with older people who represent a variety of ethnic backgrounds.

Legler, Henry. _How to Make the Rest of Your Life the Best of Your Life_. Simon and Schuster. New York, New York. 1967.

Aids are offered to achieve self discovery of interests and activities which best suit individual needs.

Merrill, Toni. _Activities for the Aged and Infirm: A Handbook for the Untrained Worker_. Charles C. Thomas. Springfield, Illois. 1967.

Detailed instructions for those interested in organizing and implementing activity programs for the aged and infirm.

______________. _Social Clubs for the Aging_. Charles C. Thomas. Springfield, Illinois. 1973.

A simple guideline for untrained leaders who direct group activities for old people; describes approximately 550 club activities.

Older Americans: The Unrealized Audience for the Arts. Center for Arts Administration. University of Wisconsin-Madison. Madison, Wisconsin. 1976.

A monograph that gives the results of a national survey about the aged as a potential arts audience. It also discusses ways to develop this audience, and offers selected programs that are directed to older persons.

Preston, Newell T. New Life for Retired Men. Exposition Press. New York, New York. 1968.

Discussion of the Retired Men's Club of Needham, Massachusetts, and solutions the club offered to leisure time boredom.

Recreation and Aging. Proceedings of Institutes for Professional Leadership in Recreation, 1967-1968. California Commission on Aging. Sacramento, California. 1968.

The institutes, which were held at the University of Southern California at San Francisco State College, were designed to provide professional recreation leadership an opportunity to obtain results of research on various aspects of aging. The goal was to achieve enriched recreation programs for older people.

Recreation and Creative Activity Program in a Senior Citizens Housing Development. Cathedral Foundation. Jacksonville, Florida. 1971.

A review of method and procedures suitable for surveying recreation needs of the aged. The use of volunteers is suggested in making such surveys.

Scholer, Elmer A., and McClain, Martha D. A Selected Bibliography on Camping and Recreation for the Aging and Aged. Institute of Gerontology. University of Iowa. Iowa City, Iowa. 1968.

An annotated bibliography.

Simone, Anne W. The New Years: A New Middle Age. Alfred A. Knopf. New York, New York. 1968.

A major thesis is that people seek creative work, which is aided by the fact that intelligence shows no impairment with age.

Snook, Leslie. Gardening for the Elderly and Handicapped. Pan Books. London, England. 1968.

Explanation of gardening techniques which may be mastered even by wheel-chair patients.

Stevens, Ardis (Editor). Fun is Therapeutic. Charles C. Thomas. Springfield, Illinois. 1972.

Book to help therapeutic recreation leaders; leaders in the field of recreation are the sources for information offered.

Sunderland, Jaqueline Tippett. Older Americans and the Arts: A Human Equation. Published by the National Center for Older Americans and the Arts, NCOA and the John F. Kennedy Center for the Performing Arts. National Council on the Aging. Washington, D. C. 1973.

A monograph encouraging active participation by older persons in all phases of the arts. Gives background information, suggested community action, resources, and a bibliography.

Talking Books and the Aging. National Council on the Aging. Washington, D. C. 1973.

A brochure describing the use that can be made of talking books and cassettes prepared for older, blind and disabled persons, and their availability to both individuals and groups.

Time on Our Hands: The "Problem" of Leisure. The Ethel Percy Andrus Gerontology Center. University of Southern California. Los Angeles, California.

A monograph suggesting guidelines for implementation of more effective programs for older persons during their uncommitted hours.

Vickery, Florence E. Creative Programming for Older Adults: A Leadership Training Guide. Association Press. New York, New York. 1972.

A book which provides information about physical, social and psychological changes accompanying the normal aging process; calls attention to the leadership potential of the elderly; and offers practical approaches to creative and enriched programming for the aged. Can be used either as a text or a resource.

REHABILITATION

Boudreault, Marie-France, et al. _To Live With Dignity_. Institute of Gerontology. University of Michigan. Ann Arbor, Michigan. 1975.

One of the series "Resources in Aging," which tells the story of a group of physically and mentally impaired older persons in a mental hospital, and their participation in a milieu therapy program.

Bright, Ruth. _Music in Geriatric Care_. St. Martin's Press. New York, New York. 1972.

A description of innovative use of music with older patients who are confused, disoriented and withdrawn.

Coordinated Activity Programs for the Aged: A How-To-Do-It Manual. American Hospital Association. Chicago, Illinois. 1975.

A tested activity program is the basis for this manual which is designed for use in nursing homes and homes for the aged. Intended primarily for activity directors, it includes organization, administration, therapeutic specialties, use of volunteers, and other topics.

Coons, Dorothy H., et al. _A Therapeutic Milieu for Geriatric Patients_. Institute of Gerontology. University of Michigan. Ann Arbor, Michigan. 1969.

Report on a rehabilitation program for geriatric mental patients in a state hospital.

Cull, John G., and Hardy, Richard E. (Editors). _The Neglected Older American: Social and Rehabilitative Services_. Charles C. Thomas. Springfield, Illinois. 1973.

Exploration of the problems and needs of the elderly and suggested solutions.

DeVries, Herbert A. _Vigor Regained. A Simple, Proven Home Program for Restoring Fitness and Vitality_. Prentice-Hall, Inc. Englewood Cliffs, New Jersey. 1974.

An exercise program developed by the author after years of research; describes appropriate and safe ways in which to maintain physical health during the latter years of life through exercise and a home physical fitness program.

Griffith, Valerie Eaton. A Stroke in the Family: A Manual of Home Therapy. Dell Publishing Company. New York, New York. 1970.

A detailed sequential rehabilitation program for family use in the home for care and treatment of individuals who have had a stroke or suffered brain injury.

Hawker, M. Geriatrics for Physiotherapists and the Allied Professions. Faber and Faber. London, England. 1974.

Practical considerations are covered for the treatment and care of elderly patients, which are applicable to physical therapists, occupational therapists and others in allied health fields.

Kaminsky, M. What's Inside You, It Shines Out of You. Horizon Press. New York, New York. 1974.

A poet writes about poetry therapy for the aged. Recorded poetry therapy sessions are included as well as an anthology of poetry written by the aged.

Leutenegger, Ralph R. Patient Care and Rehabilitation of Communication-Impaired Adults. Charles C. Thomas. Springfield, Illinois. 1975.

The book is designed for both professionals and others involved in the rehabilitation and care of aging persons. The author deals with aging change and team care as well as with specific communications disabilities.

Long, Janet M. Caring For and Caring About Elderly People. American Health Care Association. Washington, D. C. (N.D.)

A book devoted to rehabilitative techniques for elderly patients with medical conditions, such as cancer and arthritis.

May, Elizabeth E., et al. Independent Living for the Handicapped and Elderly. Houghton Mifflin Company. Boston, Massachusetts. 1974.

This book is directed to the physically limited population, but offers many helps to those who work with them. Special sections are devoted to the elderly handicapped. It is simply written, profusely illustrated and has an appendix of information and instructions.

Rathbone, Josephine L., and Lucas, Carol. Recreation in Total Rehabilitation. Charles C. Thomas. Springfield, Illinois. 1970.

Discussion of recreation programs tried by the authors which seem effective with patients; written for administrators, students, social workers, nurses, recreational and occupational therapists, and families of rehabilitation patients.

Resource Materials for Communicative Problems of Older Persons. American Speech and Hearing Association. 9030 Old Georgetown Road. Washington, D. C. 20014. 1975.

An annotated bibliography of materials about hearing, language, and speech problems prevalent among elderly persons. Designed not only for use by professionals, but also for patients and their families.

Robinson, Alice M. Remotivation Techniques: A Manual for Use in Nursing Homes. Special Project of Smith, Kline and French Laboratories. American Psychiatric Association. Washington, D. C. (N.D.)

Manual designed to assist nurses and aides in the development of remotivation programs in nursing homes.

Routh, Thomas A. Rehabilitation Counseling of the Blind. Charles C. Thomas. Springfield, Illinois. 1970.

This book includes numerous facets important in counseling, e.g., employment, mental health considerations, psychotherapy.

Rudd, Jacob L., and Margolin, Reuben J. (Editors). Maintenance Therapy for the Geriatric Patient. Charles C. Thomas. Springfield, Illinois. 1968.

Identification of the special needs of geriatric patients; explanation of methods employed in maintenance therapy for the aged, including community activity programs.

Self-Maintenance Skills. Gerontology Center. Institute for the Study of Human Development. Pennsylvania State University. University Park, Pennsylvania. 1976.

A manual designed for those working with the impaired aged in helping them maintain independent lives.

Smith, Genevieve Waples. Care of the Patient With A Stroke: A Handbook for the Patient's Family and the Nurse. Springer Publishing Company. New York, New York. 1967.

A handbook, written simply enough for a lay audience, that discusses details of care needed by a stroke patient for maximum rehabilitation.

Stephens, Louise T. (Editor). Reality Orientation: A Technique to Rehabilitating the Elderly and Brain Damaged Patient With A Moderate to Severe Degree of Disorientation. American Psychiatric Association. Washington, D. C. 1969.

A monograph analyzing reality orientation, including a discussion of technique based precepts and guidelines as well as case histories of results.

Therapeutic Recreation Annual. (Formerly Recreation in Treatment Centers). National Recreation and Park Association. National Therapeutic Recreation Society. Arlington, Virginia. Updated annually.

Discussion of the growing link between the therapeutic recreation specialist and other medical fields. This publication is compiled annually by members of the National Therapeutic Recreation Society and professionals in gerontology, medicine, and allied health fields.

Therapeutic Workshop for Older Persons. Monograph No. 5. Final Report. Jewish Vocational Service. Chicago, Illinois. 1966.

A discussion of the place of mental health practices and the use of work in treating the emotionally disturbed.

Wilson, Philip K. (Editor). Adult Fitness and Cardiac Rehabilitation. University Park Press. Baltimore, Maryland. 1975.

A resource text for those directing exercise programs for adults. Focuses primarily on the cardiovascular system.

Wolff, Kurt. The Emotional Rehabilitation of the Geriatric Patient. Charles C. Thomas. Springfield, Illinois. 1970.

A book on the relationship between treatment methods, physical health of the patient, and social factors concerning him. Considers the elderly as both hospital in-patient and out-patient. A review of long established as well as more recent approaches to prevention of illness, treatments of emotional problems and rehabilitation for the aged.

U. S. GOVERNMENT PUBLICATIONS

Art Therapy: A Bibliography. Department of Health, Education and Welfare. Superintendent of Documents. U. S. Government Printing Office. Washington, D. C. 1974.

Institute on Rehabilitation of the Aging. Proceedings. U. S. Department of Health, Education and Welfare. Social and Rehabilitation Service. Superintendent of Documents. U. S. Government Printing Office. Washington, D. C. 1968.

Recommended For Action: Disability and Rehabilitation. White House Conference on Aging. Superintendent of Documents. U. S. Government Printing Office. Washington, D. C. 1972.

RETIREMENT

Adler, Joan. The Retirement Book. William Morrow and Company, Inc. New York, New York. 1975.

A comprehensive guide for planning early retirement, including: finances, new activities, and living arrangements.

AIM's Money Management Guide to Independent Living. AIM Division. American Association of Retired Persons. Washington, D. C. 1972.

One of a series of topical monographs on planning for a successful retirement.

Arnold, Suzanne, et al. Ready or Not: A Study Manual for Retirement. Manpower Education Institute. New York, New York. 1974.

A handbook offering suggestions and guidelines for those facing retirement.

Askwith, Herbert. Your Retirement: How to Plan For It, How to Enjoy It to the Fullest. Hart Publishing Company. New York, New York. 1974.

The author writes for the person looking forward to retirement and makes suggestions and offers information designed to produce rewarding retirement years.

Atchley, Robert C. The Sociology of Retirement. Halsted Press/John Wiley and Sons. New York, New York. 1976.

The author faces the evolution of retirement as a product of industrial society.

Bowman, Donald L. How Pre-retirement Planning Works: A Guide for Program Planners. Drake University Pre-retirement Planning Center. Des Moines, Iowa. 1972.

A guide to establishing and administering pre-retirement programs.

Buckley, Joseph C. The Retirement Book. Harper and Row. New York, New York. 1974.

Topics include financial preparation, leisure and others. The philosophy expressed concerning leisure may not find consistent acceptance.

Carp, Frances M. (Editor). Retirement. Behavioral Publications, Inc. New York, New York. 1972.

An analysis of retirement based upon research findings from anthropology, economics, medicine, psychology, psychiatry and sociology.

Corrigan, B. Retire With Pride, Purpose and Pleasure. Exposition Press. Hicksville, New York. 1975.

Helpful hints on how to maintain one's standard of living into retirement. Topics covered include housing, health, legal matters, taxes, insurance, and investing.

Claiborn, William L., and Kayton, Robert. Coping With Old Age. Nelson-Hall, Inc., Publishers. Chicago, Illinois. In press.

The book is designed for an audience spanning pre-retirement and post retirement, reviewing common problems and solutions. Topics include: personal adjustment, housing, money, family and wills.

Collins, Thomas. The Complete Guide to Retirement. Prentice-Hall, Inc. Englewood Cliffs, New Jersey. 1970.

Suggestions for making retirement an easy and pleasurable experience; covers financial, legal, and health problems; change of residence, relations with children; and retirement homes.

Cooley, Leland Frederick, and Cooley, Lee Morrison. How to Avoid the Retirement Trap. Nash Publishing. Los Angeles, California. 1972.

The difficulties faced by those approaching retirement are identified; advice offered for avoiding the problems. Subjects discussed include: Social Security, Medicare, investments, retirement communities, physical and mental aging.

Corrick, Frank. Preparing for Your Retirement Years: A Question and Answer Guide Showing How to Achieve Independence by Properly Planning for Retirement. Pilot Books. New York, New York. 1972.

A planning guide for persons facing retirement; also beneficial to those in retirement.

Dickinson, Peter A. The Complete Retirement Planning Book. E. P. Dutton & Company, Inc. New York, New York. 1976.

A guidebook to retirement which advises the retiree in the areas of health, finances, housing, legal matters, and leisure.

Dixon, Daniel. Can You Retire? Some Thoughts About the Individual, Administrative and Economic Aspects of Retirement. Pergamon Press. New York, New York. 1968.

General discussion of income, health, companionship, and status problems confronting those nearing retirement.

Draper, Jean E., et al. Work Attitudes and Retirement Adjustment. The University of Wisconsin. Graduate School of Business. Bureaus of Business Research and Service. Madison, Wisconsin. 1967.

Exploration of attitudes toward work, retirement, and adjustment in retirement.

Duffus, R. L. Adventure in Retirement. W. W. Norton & Co., Inc. New York, New York. 1965.

Suggestions for retirement activities.

Geist, Harold. The Psychological Aspects of Retirement. Charles C. Thomas. Springfield, Illinois. 1968.

Coverage includes psychological and physiological aging, a brief history of retirement and pension plans, and presents some of the problems associated with retirement.

Greene, Mark R., et al. Early Retirement: A Survey of Company Policies and Retirees Experiences. University of Oregon. Graduate School of Management and Business. Eugene, Oregon. 1969.

A pilot survey of approximately 200 companies and 1,000 persons who retired early; discusses company policies for retirement with an overview of the retirees in terms of finances, health, and the relationship between planned retirement and later adjustment.

Hansen, Percy M. Never Too Late to be Young. Fell Press. New York, New York. 1966.

Arguments given against the forced retirement system and taxation of the younger generation to pay for services to the aged.

Havighurst, Robert J., et al. (Editors). Adjustment to Retirement. Van Gorcum & Company. Assen, The Netherlands. 1970.

A cross-national study of adjustment problems in retirement.

Hepner, Harry Walker. Retirement: A Time to Live Anew; A Practical Guide to Managing Your Retirement. McGraw-Hill Book Company. New York, New York. 1969.

A general discussion of physical, psychological, and economic aspects of retirement with one chapter devoted to housing and locations for retirees.

Herold, Sister Duchesne. New Life: Preparation of Religious for Retirement. The Catholic Hospital Association. St. Louis, Missouri. 1974.

Author shares with the religious community her knowledge of positive attitudes toward retirement.

Hersey, Jean, and Hersey, Robert. Change in the Wind. Charles Scribner's Sons. New York, New York. 1972.

Sequel to These Rich Years, which described experiences of a newly retired couple; Change in the Wind discusses a later time in their lives when there had been geographic relocation; a look at the problems and joys of a seemingly affluent older couple.

____________________________. These Rich Years, A Journal of Retirement. Charles Scribner's Sons. New York, New York. 1969.

Reflections on a couple's first three years of retirement.

Heusinkveld, Helen, and Musson, Noverre Best Places to Live When You Retire: A National Directory of Retirement Residences. Frederick Fell, Inc. New York, New York. 1969.

Needs of retirees discussed; information on available types of residences and factors to consider in selecting a place to live.

Hills, L. Rust. How to Retire at Forty-one: Or Dropping Out of the Rat Race Without Going Down the Drain. Doubleday & Company. Garden City, New York. 1973.

A humorous treatment of a serious subject. The underlying thesis is that retirement is a vocation to be structured to achieve usefulness and resulting self-respect.

How Pre-Retirement Planning Works: Results and Findings in a Three-Year Demonstration. Drake University Pre-Retirement Planning Center. Des Moines, Iowa. 1970.

The purpose of this program was to test the effectiveness of pre-retirement counseling; includes fringe benefits, employment after retirement, investments, leisure time activities, psychological aspects of retirement, etc. A continuing evaluation follow-up of the program effectiveness was conducted.

Hoyt, Murray. Creative Retirement: Planning the Best Years Yet. Garden Way Publishers. Charlotte, Vermont. 1974.

Book designed to assist the planning ahead for retirement, giving attention to individual needs and desires.

Hunter, Woodrow W. Preparation for Retirement (Third Edition). Institute of Gerontology. Ann Arbor, Michigan. 1976.

A new edition of the informative guidelines for persons anticipating retirement. Covers a broad scope of pertinent topics.

Ingraham, Mark H. My Purpose Holds. Winchell. Philadelphia, Pennsylvania. 1974.

This book presents the results of a TIAA-CREF survey of its annuitants. Its purpose is to give a personal view of retirement through individual reactions and experiences. The findings demonstrate the vastness of individual response to retirement.

Kelly, Philip J. Second Wind: Handbook for Happy Retirement. McIlvaine Publishing Company. Hendersonville, North Carolina. 1972.

This book deals with realities concerning life after retirement. The author draws upon ten years of experience as a retiree, and offers suggestions designed for people over fifty.

Mathiasen, Geneva (Editor). Criteria for Retirement. G. P. Putnam's Sons. New York, New York. 1973.

Criteria other than age considered useful in determining retirement policies. Discusses social needs, economic problems, responsibilities of employers, workers, unions, and government in relation to retirement.

Margolius, Sidney. Your Personal Guide to Successful Retirement. Random House. New York, New York. 1969.

A readable, practical guide written in modified outline format. Covers a broad range of topics.

Mitchell, William L. (Editor). Preparation for Retirement. American Association of Retired Persons. Washington, D. C. 1968.

A guide for those engaged in the development and administration of pre-retirement programs, it offers information on types of programs, group meeting topics, program content, program evaluation, and post-retirement services.

Olmstead, Alan H. Threshold: The First Days of Retirement. Harper and Row, Publishers. New York, New York. 1975.

Written in diary format. The author recounts the first seven months of his retirement, dealing reflectively with pleasures and disappointments on his new phase of life. Interesting and also encouraging.

Orbach, Harold L., et al. Trends in Early Retirement. Occasional Papers in Gerontology. Institute of Gerontology. University of Michigan. Ann Arbor, Michigan. 1969.

Compilation of papers originally presented in hearings before the U. S. Senate Special Committee on Aging relating trends in early retirement among industrial and civil service workers to current political and economic debate.

Otte, Elmer. Rehearse Before You Retire. Second Edition. Retirement Research. Appleton-Century-Crofts. New York, New York. 1973.

Suggestions for planning purposeful activity in the retirement years.

__________ Retirement Rehearsal Guidebook. Pictorial, Inc. Indianapolis, Indiana. Revised, 1974.

Information which every pre-retiree should know plus a battery of questions to get one started thinking about his retirement. Provides space for recording vital information pertinent to one's retirement.

__________ Welcome Retirement. Concordia Publishing House. St. Louis, Missouri. 1974.

The author, now retired for twelve years, writes about the problems and offers advice he has followed in adjustments to retirement.

Pollard, Lu Lu. Retirement - Black and White. Exposition Press, Inc. New York, New York. 1973.

A black author takes a look at the special retirement problems of the low income black elderly. Racial differences and commonalities are also considered.

Pre-retirement Counseling, Retirement Adjustment, and the Older Employee. College of Business Administration. University of Oregon. Eugene, Oregon. 1969.

A study of factors related to the effectiveness of the older worker, resistance to retirement, and adjustment in retirement.

Pre-Retirement and the Older Worker. Summary of Proceedings of Conference Sponsored by Pennsylvania Office of Aging. Administrative Management Society. Carlisle Area Personnel Association and National Council on Aging. National Council on the Aging. Washington, D. C. 1975.

The papers presented at the conference designed to exchange knowledge and experience and to encourage establishment of comprehensive pre-retirement programs.

Pre-Retirement Planning. National Council on the Aging. Washington, D. C. Revised periodically.

An annotated bibliography.

"Retirement." _The Gerontologist_, Volume II, No. 1, Part 1. The Gerontological Society. Washington, D. C. Spring, 1971.

An issue of _The Gerontologist_ devoted solely to retirement; includes pre-planning, leisure time participation, institutional services, community resources and service to facilitate independent living.

Retirement Income. National Council on the Aging. Washington, D. C. Revised periodically.

An annotated bibliography.

Retirement Planning: Selected References. Gerontology Center. Institute for the Study of Human Development. Pennsylvania State University. University Park, Pennsylvania. 1975.

A bibliography of more than 1,000 articles and books on retirement and pre-retirement planning.

Retirement and Retirement Planning. National Council on the Aging. Washington, D. C. Revised periodically.

an annotated bibliography.

Smith, Patricia C., et al. _The Measurement of Satisfaction in Work and Retirement: A Strategy for the Study of Attitudes_. Rand McNally and Company. Chicago, Illinois. 1969.

Description of the development of measurement techniques, with information on their use and interpretation.

Streib, Gordon F., and Schneider, Clement J. _Retirement in American Society: Impact and Process_. Cornell University Press. Ithaca, New York. 1971.

A report and analysis of a nationwide, large-scale longitudinal study of retirement undertaken by the Cornell Study of Occupational Retirement. Older workers were first contacted while still employed and followed up four times during the next six years.

Sunshine, John. How to Enjoy Your Retirement. AMACOM. New York, New York. 1974.

Oriented primarily toward the male, this book offers suggestions to facilitate adjustment in retirement. Appendices include helpful directory information for retirees.

Ware, George W. The New Guide to Happy Retirement. Crown Publishers, Inc. New York, New York. 1968.

General discussion on how to enjoy retirement; includes financial management, change of residence, and other topics.

U. S. GOVERNMENT PUBLICATIONS

Federal Role in Encouraging Preretirement Counseling and New Work Lifetime Patterns, The. Hearings before the Subcommittee on Retirement and the Individual. Ninety-first Congress. U. S. Senate. First Session. Special Committee on Aging. Superintendent of Documents. U. S. Government Printing Office. Washington, D. C. 1970.

Gallaway, Lowell E. The Retirement Decision: An Exploratory Essay. Research Report No. 9. Superintendent of Documents. U. S. Government Printing Office. Washington, D. C. 1965.

Handbook on Retirement Services for Army Personnel and Their Families. U. S. Government Printing Office. Washington, D. C. 1975.

Irelan, Lola M., et al. Almost 65: Baseline Data from the Retirement History Study. U. S. Department of Health, Education and Welfare. Social Security Administration. Office of Research and Statistics. Research Report No. 49. HEW Publication No. (SSA) 76-11806. Superintendent of Documents. U. S. Government Printing Office. Washington, D. C. 1976.

Parnes, Herbert S., et al. The Pre-Retirement Years. U. S. Department of Labor, Manpower Administration. Manpower Research Monograph No. 15. U. S. Government Printing Office. Washington, D. C.

Volume 1. 1970.
Volume 2. 1970.
Volume 3. 1973.
Volume 4. 1975.

Planning for the Later Years. U. S. Social Security Administration. Superintendent of Documents. U. S. Government Printing Office. Washington, D. C. 1967.

Retirement and the Individual. Hearings Before the Subcommittee on Retirement and the Individual of the Special Committee on Aging. United States Senate. Ninety-First Congress. First Session. Superintendent of Documents. U. S. Government Printing Office. Washington, D. C. June 7-8, 1967.

Retirement Roles and Activities. White House Conference on Aging. Superintendent of Documents. U. S. Government Printing Office. Washington, D. C. 1972.

You, The Law, and Retirement. Administration on Aging. AOA Publication No. 800. Superintendent of Documents. U. S. Government Printing Office. Washington, D. C. 1965.

SAFETY

Furniture Requirements for Older People. National Council on the Aging. Washington, D. C. 1963.

Although an old publication, this small volume remains a valuable resource on appropriate furniture for older persons, including design and the relationship of suitable furniture to health and safety. Includes recommendations for designers, manufacturers and purchasers.

Koncelik, Joseph A. Considerate Design and the Aging: Review Article With a Selected and Annotated Bibliography. Council of Planning Librarians. Monticello, Illinois. 1972.

A compilation of publications in which criteria are established for design of products and building interiors to benefit older persons. Reviews literature and offers a bibliography.

Life Safety Code, 1973. National Fire Protection Association. Boston, Massachusetts. 1973.

Chapter 10 is concerned with institutions and protection of occupants.

Proceedings of National Conference on the Aging Driver. Health and Safety Associations. Morton Grove, Illinois. 1974.

Report on a meeting sponsored by the American Medical Association and the American Association of Motor Vehicle Administrators. Includes papers presented and recommendations that were made.

Ranney, M. W. Fire Retardant Building Products and Coatings. Noyes Data Corporation. Park Ridge, New Jersey. 1970.

Title self-explanatory.

Small, Arnold M.(Editor). Safety For the Elderly. The Ethel Percy Andrus Gerontology Center. University of Southern California. Los Angeles, California. 1975.

A bibliography.

U. S. GOVERNMENT PUBLICATIONS

Caravaty, Raymond D., and Haviland, David S. *Life Safety From Fire: A Guide for Housing the Elderly*. Superintendent of Documents. U. S. Government Printing Office. Washington, D. C. 1968.

Errors in Fire Safety Inspections of Nursing Homes. Hearing before a Subcommittee of the Committee on Government Operations. House of Representatives. Ninety-Third Congress. Second Session. U. S. Government Printing Office. Washington, D. C. June, 1974.

Fire Safety in Highrise Buildings for the Elderly. Subcommittee on Housing for the Elderly. Special Committee on Aging. Ninety-Third Congress. First Session. U. S. Senate. Superintendent of Documents. U. S. Government Printing Office. Washington, D. C. 1973.

Flammable Fabrics and Other Fire Hazards to Older Americans: Hearing. Special Committee on Aging. Ninety-Second Congress. First Session. U. S. Senate. Superintendent of Documents. U. S. Government Printing Office. Washington, D. C. 1972.

Lewis, Dorothea J., and Winsor, Richard J. *Handle Yourself With Care*. Administration on Aging. U. S. Department of Health, Education and Welfare. U. S. Government Printing Office. Washington, D. C. 1969.

SENIOR CENTERS

Booth, F. Estelle. Reaching Out to the Hard-to-Reach Older Person. Second Edition. San Francisco Senior Center. San Francisco, California. 1969.

Information is given on the operation of a senior center with ways suggested to involve unmotivated old people.

Directory of Senior Centers and Clubs: A National Resource, 1974. National Council on Aging. Washington, D. C. 1974.

A listing of almost 4900 centers and clubs throughout the United States, including, sponsors, services provided, accomodation for wheelchairs, and other related information.

Expanding Senior Center Services to the Impaired Elderly. National Council on the Aging. Washington, D. C. 1975.

This is a practical guide for those in senior centers who are working with the elderly who have physical, visual or hearing impairments.

First National Conference of Senior Centers. National Council on the Aging. Washington, D. C. 1964.

Describes the senior center as a comprehensive, activity-oriented agency.

Fowler, Talmadge D. Alternatives to the Single Site Center. The National Council on the Aging, Inc. Washington, D. C. 1974.

A description of how senior center networks with satellites or mobile units scattered throughout the community might be developed as a way to expand services.

Jacobs, Bella. Involving Men - A Challenge for Senior Centers. National Council on the Aging. Washington, D. C. 1974.

An examination of problems encountered in encouraging men to participate in senior centers. Discusses characteristics of older men that affect program development, criteria for effective programming, role of staff, motivation, the handicapped and minorities.

Jacobs, Bella. (Editor). Senior Centers: Options and Actions. The National Council on the Aging. Washington, D. C. 1975.

Proceedings of the Ninth National Conference of Senior Centers. Topics included: options and functions for centers, alternative models, techniques for planning and evaluation, services for impaired and homebound elderly, among others.

____________________. Senior Centers: Realizing our Potentials. National Council on Aging. Washington, D. C. 1975.

Proceedings of Eighth National Conference of Senior Centers in which the methods and resources to meet older peoples' needs are examined. Covers a broad range of topics.

______________(Editor). Social Action: Expanding Role for Senior Centers. The National Council on the Aging, Inc. Washington, D. C. 1974.

The focus of this monograph is upon the senior center as an appropriate vehicle for involving the elderly in social action on their own behalf. Divided into three parts, it discusses the concept of social action, mechanisms to facilitate the process, and constraints within which social action operates.

______________(Editor). Working With the Impaired Elderly. National Council on the Aging, Inc. Washington, D. C. 1976.

Basic information and guidelines for senior center practitioners and others working with the impaired elderly.

Jordan, Joe J. Senior Center Facilities: An Architect's Evaluation of Building Design, Equipment and Furnishings. National Council on Aging, Inc. Washington, D. C. 1975.

An examination of nine centers considered to be good examples of effective center facilities. Defines problems to be avoided in planning, gives floor plans and other illustrations.

Leanse, Joyce, and Wagner, Sara B. Senior Centers: A Report of Senior Group Programs in America. National Council on the Aging, Inc. Washington, D. C. 1975.

This is a report on the findings from a survey of 30 senior centers which covers programs, and information on users and non-users.

Maxwell, Jean. Centers for Older People: Guide for Programs and Facilities. National Council on the Aging. Washington, D. C. 1962. Reprinted 1973.

A basic guide for community planners, architects, board members and professional staff of multipurpose Senior Centers. An old reference which maintains current value as a reference.

Multi-Purpose Senior Center: A Model Community Action Program, The. (Revised Edition). The National Council on the Aging, Inc. Washington, D. C. 1972.

A monograph which offers practical guidelines for organizing a senior center.

Participation of the Elderly Poor in Senior Centers. The National Council on the Aging, Inc. Washington, D. C. 1970.

A monograph describing the organization and operation of senior centers in both rural and urban areas in a way to bring aged persons back into the social life of the community.

Planning Today for Tomorrow's OlderPeople. National Council on the Aging, Inc. Third National Conference of Senior Centers. National Council on the Aging. Washington, D. C. 1966.

A book offering suggestions on how center leaders can develop new ideas and keep programs current with changing times. Experiences of twenty agencies with programming, management, public relations, and other topics are discussed.

Projections for Tomorrow - Proceedings of the 10th National Conference of Senior Centers. National Institute of Senior Centers. Publications Department. The National Council on the Aging. Washington, D. C. 1976.

A collection of papers covering a variety of subjects, which were presented at the conference.

Pollak, Otto, et al. Utilization Study of a Senior Citizens Center. Weinstein Geriatric Center of the Sidney Hillman Medical Center. Philadelphia, Pennsylvania. 1970.

Utilization study of a management-union senior recreational center. Reasons for use and non-use are studied.

Selected Bibliography of NCOA Publications Concerning Senior Centers. National Institute of Senior Centers. National Council on the Aging. Washington, D. C. 1971.

A 28-page topical index of NCOA publications on senior centers, covering the period 1961-1970.

Senior Centers: A Guide to Planning, Design and Operation. National Council on the Aging, Inc. Washington, D. C. 1975.

Guidelines for organizations and agencies initiating or expanding senior center facilities and operations.

Senior Centers: A Focal Point for Delivery of Services to Older People. National Council on the Aging, Inc. Washington, D. C. 1972.

Four papers delivered at NCOA regional meetings which outline the components of a multipurpose center and innovative program ideas.

Senior Center and the Great Society, The. National Council on the Aging. Second National Conference of Senior Centers. National Council on the Aging. Washington, D. C. 1965.

An older publication in which leading authorities examine the role of the senior center in relation to poverty, racial barriers and early retirement. Has historical value.

Senior Centers Today: New Opportunities, New Challenges. National Council on the Aging's Fourth National Conference of Senior Centers. National Council on the Aging. Washington, D. C. 1967.

An evaluation of accomplishments made by the center movement within the past five years with an outline of further steps needed to provide more extensive development of the senior center.

Tiven, Marjorie Bloomberg. Health Maintenance Programs in Senior Centers. National Council on the Aging. Washington, D. C. 1973.

An examination of development and implementation of preventive health programs in senior center programs. Topics include: needs, type services, organization and staffing, financing. Consideration given to minority groups, and community resources.

Wain, Jack. Handcraft Cooperatives: New Thrust in Senior Center Programming. National Council on the Aging. Washington, D. C. 1973.

Directions for organizing and operating a handcraft cooperative, including incorporation, funding, financial management, production, quality control and marketing. A bibliography is included.

Wilson, Lola (Editor). Report: Training Institute for Directors of Senior Centers. Canadian Council on Social Development. Ottawa, Ontario, Canada. 1972.

A training program to expand knowledge base for center directors. Provides outlet for exchange of ideas and experience, and to encourage greater involvement of older persons in center operations and programming.

Wolfson, Alice D. (Editor). Challenges Facing Senior Centers in the 1970's. National Council on the Aging. New York, New York. 1969.

A report of the Fifth National Conference of Senior Centers. Includes material on the roles and functions of senior centers, emphasizing minorities, the hard-to-reach, and those with deteriorating conditions.

Working With the Impaired Elderly. National Institute of Senior Centers. Publications Department. National Council on the Aging. Washington, D. C. 1976.

These guidelines for senior center programs for impaired elderly persons include: the integration of persons physically disabled; socialization for the visually handicapped; speech and hearing rehabilitation techniques; and working with those suffering mental deterioration.

SEX AND THE ELDERLY

Birren, James E. (Editor). Sexuality and Aging. The Ethel Percy Andrus Gerontology Center. University of Southern California. Los Angeles, California. 1975.

A bibliography.

Burnside, Irene M. Sexuality and Aging. Ethel Percy Andrus Gerontology Center. University of Southern California. Los Angeles, California. 1975.

An overview of current thinking on the topic of aging and sex as viewed by biologists, physicians, social psychologists, nurses, and social workers.

Butler, Robert N., and Lewis, Myrna. Sex After Sixty. Harper and Row. New York, New York. 1976.

Coverage includes both physical and emotional aspects of sex in later life, as well as attitudes in society based upon role assignment to the elderly.

Dickinson, Peter. The Fires of Autumn: Sexual Activity in the Middle and Later Years. Drake Publishers. New York, New York. 1974.

A work devoted to the psychological, attitudinal and physical sexual problems found most commonly among middle-aged and elderly persons.

Johnson, Warren R. Sex Education and Counseling of Special Groups, The Mentally and Physically Handicapped, Ill and Elderly. Charles C. Thomas. Springfield, Illinois. 1975.

Title self-explanatory.

Felstein, Ivor. Sex in Later Life. Penguin Books, Inc. Baltimore, Maryland. 1974.

Sexual behavior is considered in the light of longer life expectancy. An attempt is made to answer basic questions regarding the impact of social expectations and physical changes in sexual behavior in old age.

Kirkendall, Lester A., and Rubin, Isadore. Sexuality and the Life Cycle. Human Sciences Press. New York, New York. 1970.

An examination of how individuals develop and manifest sexual feeling and behavior throughout the life cycle.

Marcus, Irwin M., and Francis, John J. (Editors). Masturbation from Infancy to Senescence. International Universities Press. New York, New York. 1975.

Written by physicians for physicians. A number of contributors treat the subject and express various points of view, with emphasis upon psychoanalytic ramifications.

Peterson, James A., and Payne, Barbara. Love in the Later Years. Association Press. New York, New York. 1975.

The central focus of this book is love, marriage, and sex in the later years of life. Topics such as economics and retirement planning are discussed, especially as they relate to emotional and love relationships among the aged.

Rubin, Isadore. Sexual Life After Sixty. Basic Books. New York, New York. 1965.

Study of sex life among older persons.

____________. Sexual Life in the Later Years. Behavioral Publications, Inc. New York, New York. 1970.

A discussion of the importance of increasing the understanding of sexuality and the need for sexual expression in the later years. Physical and emotional aspects of aging are considered.

Rubin, Herman H., and Newman, Benjamin W. Active Sex After Sixty. Arco Publishing Company, Inc. New York, New York. 1970.

Recommendations and advice to those interested in maintaining an active and satisfying sexual life into old age.

Scheingold, Lee D., and Wagner, Nathaniel N. Sound Sex and the Aging Heart. Behavioral Publications, Inc. New York, New York. 1974.

Based upon empirical research and clinical experience, this book deals with the psychological and physiological aspects of aging as they relate to cardiac conditions and sexual activities.

Sexuality in the Later Years of Life. Institute of Gerontology. University of Michigan. Ann Arbor, Michigan. 1975.

Annotated bibliography on topic specified.

Van der Berghe, Pierre L. Age and Sex in Human Societies: A Bio-Social Perspective. Wadsworth Publishing Company. Belmont, California. 1973.

Sexuality is discussed in the context of age and cultural influences.

Wikler, Revy, and Grey, Peg Savage. Sex and the Senior Citizen. Fell Publishing Company. New York, New York. 1968.

A report on real life experiences of old people and how they deal with sex in later life.

SOCIAL SECURITY

Altmeyer, Arthur J. The Formative Years of Social Security. University of Wisconsin Press. Madison, Wisconsin. 1966.

Background information leading to passage of the Social Security Act and historical data on the program during its growth and development from 1934 to 1954.

Analysis and Partial Legislative History of Title II of Public Law 92-603 (H.R.1), "The Social Security Amendments of 1972," An. Government Relations Department. American Nursing Home Association. Washington, D. C. 1973.

A manual of pertinent information relative to Social Security amendments of particular interest to those concerned with nursing home care programs and others working in areas affected by revision of the Social Security Laws.

Cohen, Wilbur J. Social Security - The First Thirty-Five Years. Occasional Papers in Gerontology. Institute of Gerontology. University of Michigan. Ann Arbor, Michigan. 1972.

A review of the past and of present Social Security pensions, and a look toward the future of the Social Security System in the United States.

__________ and Friedman, Milton. Social Security Universal or Selective. American Enterprise Institute for Public-Policy Research. Washington, D. C. 1972.

Wilbur Cohen, one of the architects of the Social Security System, considers some vital issues of the system with Chicago economist, Milton Friedman.

Lubove, Roy. The Struggle for Social Security, 1900-1935. Harvard University Press. Cambridge, Massachusetts. 1968.

A comprehensive review of the evolution of Social Security in the United States up to the New Deal.

Melemed, Brina B. Title XX of the Social Security Act: A Resource for Serving the Needs of Older People. The National Council on the Aging. Washington, D. C. 1976.

The first report of the NCOA Title XX Assessment Project, this monograph summarizes the legislation and regulations and is designed to encourage better utilization of the Title XX program for services to older persons.

Munnell, Alicia H. The Effect of Social Security on Personal Savings. Ballinger Publishing Company. Cambridge, Massachusetts. 1974.

The author has attempted to show the dual effects of social security upon savings, one positive and one negative. Interesting points of emphasis are made, but certain omissions in developing the thesis appear to have pertinence.

Old-Age, Survivors and Disability Insurance and Medicare Programs. Advisory Council on Social Security. Baltimore, Maryland. 1973.

This publication up-dates the provisions of old-age, survivors, disability and Medicare programs to time of issue, and gives pertinent data on them.

Pechman, Joseph A., et al. Social Security: Perspectives for Reform. The Brookings Institute. Washington, D. C. 1968.

Recommendations for supplements to the Social Security System in the form of negative income tax or some other reformed system of public assistance.

Rhee, H. A. Human Ageing and Retirement. General Secretariat. International Social Security Association. Geneva, Switzerland. 1974.

This study recognized the need for expanded attention to Social Security on a world-wide basis. The premise considered is that aging and retirement affect both individual and society, as well as being affected by society. Similarly, Social Security needs to look outside itself into the community for answers to problems. Wide knowledge gaps are described as the failure of Social Security and gerontology to find a meeting ground.

U. S. GOVERNMENT PUBLICATIONS

Estimating Your Social Security Retirement Check. Social Security Administration. DHEW Publication No. (SSA) 75-10047. U. S. Department of Health, Education, and Welfare. U. S. Government Printing Office. Washington, D. C. 1975.

Future Directions in Social Security. Hearings before the Special Committee on Aging. United States Senate. U. S. Government Printing Office. Washington, D. C. Parts 1-25. 1973-1976.

Future Directions in Social Security - Unresolved Issues: An Interim Staff Report. Special Committee on Aging. United States Senate. Ninety-third Congress. Superintendent of Documents. U. S. Government Printing Office. Washington, D. C. March, 1975.

Health Insurance for the Aged. Bureau of Health Insurance. Social Security Administration. U. S. Department of Health, Education and Welfare. Social Security Publication No. 69-59 (11-73). Superintendent of Documents. U. S. Government Printing Office. Washington, D. C. 1973.

History of the Provisions of Old-Age, Survivors, Disability, and Health Insurance. U. S. Department of Health, Education and Welfare. Social Security Administration. Reprinted from the Social Security Bulletin, Annual Statistical Supplement, 1970. DHEW Publication No. (SSA) 73-11700. Superintendent of Documents. U. S. Government Printing Office. Washington, D. C. 1972.

OASDI Digest: The Cash Benefit Provisions of the Old-Age, Survivors, and Disability Insurance System. U. S. Department of Health. Education and Welfare. Social Security Administration. Superintendent of Documents. U. S. Government Printing Office. Washington, D. C. 1974.

Preliminary Findings from the Survey of New Beneficiaries. U. S. Department of Health, Education and Welfare. Social Security Administration. Office of Research and Statistics. Report No. 5. Washington, D. C. August, 1971.

Schiltz, Michael E. Public Attitudes Toward Social Security, 1935-1965. Research Report No. 33. Superintendent of Documents. U. S. Government Printing Office. Washington, D. C. 1970.

Smith, Richard T., and Lilienfeld, Abraham M. Social Security Disability Program: An Evaluation Study, The. U. S. Department of Health, Education and Welfare. Social Security Administration. Office of Research and Statistics. Research Report No. 39. Publication No. (SSA) 72-11801. Superintendent of Documents. U. S. Government Printing Office. Washington, D. C. 1971.

Social Security Amendments of 1972. Committee on Finance. Ninety-Second Congress. U. S. Senate. Superintendent of Documents. U. S. Government Printing Office. Washington, D. C. 1972.

Social Security Handbook, Retirement Insurance, Survivors Insurance, Disability Insurance, Health Insurance, Black Lung Benefits, Supplemental Security Income. Fifth Edition. Social Security Administration. Department of Health, Education and Welfare. Superintendent of Documents. U. S. Government Printing Office. Washington, D. C. 1974.

Social Security Programs Throughout the World, 1969. U. S. Department of Health, Education and Welfare. Social Security Administration. Office of Research and Statistics. Superintendent of Documents. U. S. Government Printing Office. Washington, D. C. 1970.

Social Security Programs Throughout the World, 1975. U. S. Department of Health, Education and Welfare. Social Security Administration. Office of Research and Statistics. Research Report No. 48. Superintendent of Documents. U. S. Government Printing Office. Washington, D. C. 1975.

Social Security Programs in the United States. Social Security Administration. Superintendent of Documents. U. S. Government Printing Office. Washington, D. C. 1973.

Social Security Rulings on Federal Old-Age, Survivors, Disability, Health Insurance, and Miner's Benefits: Cumulative Bulletin 1972. Social Security Administration. U. S. Department of Health, Education and Welfare. Superintendent of Documents. U. S. Government Printing Office. Washington, D. C. 1973.

Women and Social Security: Adapting to a New Era. A Working Paper Prepared by the Task Force on Women and Social Security. Special Committee on Aging. United States Senate. Ninety-fourth Congress. Superintendent of Documents. U. S. Government Printing Office. Washington, D. C. October, 1975.

Your Social Security. Social Security Administration. DHEW Publication No. (SSA) 75-10035. U. S. Department of Health, Education and Welfare. U. S. Government Printing Office. Washington, D. C. 1975.

Your Social Security, Retirement, Survivors and Disability Insurance, Medicare. U. S. Social Security Administration. Superintendent of Documents. U. S. Government Printing Office. Washington, D. C. 1971.

TRANSPORTATION

Ahrens, Robert J. Reduced Fares for Senior Citizens. Division for Senior Citizens. Department of Human Resources. Chicago, Illinois. 1970.

Description of a program developed by the Chicago Division for Senior Citizens; provides basic information and materials for cities and regional planners interested in reduction in fares to the elderly.

Falcocchio, John C., and Cantilli, Edmund J. Transportation and the Disadvantaged: The Poor, the Young, the Elderly, the Handicapped. Lexington Books. Lexington, Massachusetts. 1974.

A discussion of problems and solutions in the area of transportation for special groups in relation to employment.

Gelwicks, Louis E. Transportation and Its Influence Upon the Quality of the Older Person's Relation With the Environment. University of Southern California. Los Angeles, California. 1970.

A discussion of ways in which transportation affects the quality of life in old age.

Revis, Joseph S. Transportation for the Elderly: Action at the Local Level. National Retired Teachers Association and American Association of Retired Persons. Washington, D. C. 1974.

A paper prepared for the National Forum on Aging for Local Government Officials to provide guidance to those concerned with the transportation problem of the elderly at the local level. It offers insight regarding alternatives available, and the various ways in which transportation programs can be organized, funded and operated.

Senior Citizen Bus Transportation Project. Prince George's County, Maryland. Division of Services and Programs for the Aging. Capitol Heights, Maryland. 1971.

Manual showing how one county provides transportation for the elderly by special buses purchased and maintained for this purpose.

Transportation for the Elderly. National Council on the Aging. Washington, D. C. (Revised periodically.)

An annotated bibliography.

U. S. GOVERNMENT PUBLICATIONS

Better Transportation for our Senior Citizens. U. S. Department of Transportation. Superintendent of Documents. U. S. Government Printing Office. Washington, D. C. 1972.

Cantilli, Edmund J., et al (Editors). *Transportation and Aging*. Administration on Aging. U. S. Department of Health, Education and Welfare. DHEW Publication No. (SRS) 72-20232. Superintendent of Documents. U. S. Government Printing Office. Washington, D. C. 1971.

Older Americans and Transportation: A Crisis in Mobility. A Report by the Special Committee on Aging. United States Senate. Superintendent of Documents. U. S. Government Printing Office. Washington, D. C. 1970.

Planning Handbook: Transportation Services for the Elderly. U. S. Department of Health, Education and Welfare. Administration on Aging. Publications Office. Washington, D. C. 1976.

Public Transportation for Elderly and Handicapped. Office of Public Affairs. Urban Mass Transportation Administration. U. S. Transportation Department. Superintendent of Documents. U. S. Government Printing Office. Washington, D. C. 1971.

Recommended for Action: Transportation. White House Conference on Aging. Superintendent of Documents. U. S. Government Printing Office. Washington, D. C. 1972.

Reduced Rate Transportation for Certain Persons. Committee on Commerce. Ninety-third Congress. United States Senate. Senate Documents Room. The Capitol. Washington, D. C. 1973.

Reduced Rate Transportation for Youth, Elderly, and Handicapped. Subcommittee on Aviation. Commerce Committee. United States Senate. Ninety-third Congress. First Session. Superintendent of Documents. U. S. Government Printing Office. Washington, D. C. 1974.

Transportation and the Elderly: Problems and Progress. Hearings before the Special Committee on Aging. United States Senate. Ninety-fourth Congress. Part 5. Washington, D. C., 1975. U. S. Government Printing Office. Washington, D. C. 1976.

Transportation for the Elderly: The State of the Art. Office of Human Development. U. S. Department of Health, Education and Welfare. Washington, D. C. 1975.

Travel Barriers. U. S. Department of Transportation. Superintendent of Documents. U. S. Government Printing Office. Washington, D. C. 1970.

VOLUNTEERS

Arthur, Julietta K. Retire to Action: A Guide to Voluntary Service. Abingdon Press. Nashville, Tennessee. 1969.

Specific recommendations for remaining active and useful in retirement. Agencies and regional possibilities for service are explored.

Aves, Geraldine M. The Voluntary Worker in the Social Services. Allen and Unwin, Ltd. London, England. 1969.

British study which examines the use of voluntary workers in community organizations and government.

David, Anne. A Guide to Volunteer Services. Cornerstone Library. New York, New York. 1970.

A handbook which suggests how one might use his special talents in volunteer work.

Ewalt, Patricia L. (Editor). Mental Health Volunteers: The Expanding Role of the Volunteer in Hospital and Community Mental Health Services. Charles C. Thomas. Springfield, Illinois. 1967.

Title self explanatory.

Faunce, Frances Avery. The Nursing Home Visitor. Abingdon Press. Nashville, Tennessee. 1968.

Guidelines for the volunteer visitor; offers information on nursing home organization, and suggests ways to facilitate patient acceptance of and adjustment to the nursing home. Written by a nursing home patient.

Hand-in-Hand: Cross-Age Interactions. Girl Scouts of the U. S. A. 830 Third Avenue. New York, New York. 10022. (N.D.)

A report on the activities of the seven girl scout councils participating in this project, which is a national undertaking to involve girl scout councils with older persons.

Intergenerational Programming. The National Council on the Aging. Washington, D. C. 1975.

A training guide prepared for youth groups who work with programs for the elderly, including senior centers.

It's Good to Have a Friend. Age Center of Worcester Area. Worcester, Massachusetts. 1970.

Tips offered on establishing and operating a Friendly Visitor Program; discusses visitor relationships with aged persons and the importance of sensitivity.

Konopka, Gisela. *Group Work in the Institution: A Modern Challenge*. Revised Edition. Association Press. New York, New York. 1970.

Book written for both professional and lay readers who perform services to persons in institutions, including the elderly.

Kurtz, Harold P., and Burrows, Margaret. *Effective Use of Volunteers in Hospitals, Homes, and Agencies*. Charles C. Thomas. Springfield, Illinois. 1970.

Guidelines for the successful implementation of volunteer programs, as well as the rationale, motivation and the scope of services which can be provided by volunteers.

Manual on Volunteer Services in Homes for the Aging and Nursing Homes. Texas Association of Homes for the Aging. Austin, Texas. 1970.

A comprehensive look at volunteer services in homes for the aging and nursing homes, including lists of resources, films and bibliographies.

Older Volunteer Training Program. The Ethel Percy Andrus Gerontology Center. The University of Southern California. Los Angeles, California. (N.D.)

A position paper on issues and training models related to volunteerism. An excellent guide and resource for those planning a volunteer program.

Roberts, Nesta. Our Future Selves: Care of the Elderly. Allen and Unwin, Ltd. London, England. 1970.

A study of the development of services for the elderly, particularly the National Old People's Welfare Council of Great Britain in 1940.

Routh, Thomas A. The Volunteer and Community Agencies. Charles C. Thomas. Springfield, Illinois. 1972.

A discussion of the need for and use of volunteers in community work; applicable to all ages.

Sainer, Janet S., and Zander, Mary L. SERVE: Older Volunteers in Community Service - A New Role and a New Resource. Community Service Society of New York. New York, New York. 1971.

A comprehensive report on SERVE (Serve and Enrich Retirement by Volunteer Experience), which describes the development of a project designed to create a productive, prestigious social role for older persons.

Shenfield, Barbara, and Allen, Isobel. The Organization of Voluntary Service: A Study of Domiciliary Visiting of the Elderly by Volunteers. Political and Economic Planning. London, England. 1972.

Findings and recommendations from a study made of friendly visiting programs in England.

Stenzel, Ann K., and Feeney, Helen M. Volunteer Training and Development: A Manual for Community Groups. Seabury Press. New York, New York. 1968.

A manual emphasizing the continuous learning aspects of volunteer service.

Volunteer in Long-Term Care, The. American Hospital Association. Chicago, Illinois. 1968.

Discussion of volunteer service in long-term care facilities.

U. S. GOVERNMENT PUBLICATIONS

Kramer, Leo. Recommendations for Developing RSVP, Retired Senior Volunteer Program. Prepared for Administration on Aging. U. S. Department of Health, Education and Welfare. Superintendent of Documents. U. S. Government Printing Office. Washington, D. C. 1971.

Older Volunteers in the Peace Corps. United States Peace Corps. Washington, D. C. 1967.

Young Girl Scout - The Older American: Service to Each Other, The. U. S. Department of Health, Education and Welfare. Social and Rehabilitation Service. Administration on Aging. AOA Publication No. 169. Superintendent of Documents. U. S. Government Printing Office. Washington, D. C. 1970.

PERIODICALS

PERIODICALS

A SAMPLING OF JOURNALS, NEWSLETTERS, AND BULLETINS IN THE FIELD OF GERONTOLOGY

Aged Care and Counseling. The Haworth Press. 174 Fifth Avenue. New York, New York 10010. (Bi-monthly).

A new journal designed specifically for mental health and health care personnel who work with the elderly in a wide variety of settings.

Ageing International. International Federation on Ageing. 1909 K Street, N. W. Washington, D. C. 20049. (Quarterly).

Publication is in English, French and German. Designed to provide readers with cross-cultural information on program innovation and service delivery, applied research, aging policy developments in such organizations as WHO, ILO, and UNESCO, and news of advocacy by volunteer agencies as well as by the aged themselves.

Aging. Office of Human Development, Administration on Aging. U. S. Department of Health, Education and Welfare. Superintendent of Documents. U. S. Government Printing Office. Washington, D. C. 20402. (Monthly).

A publication largely devoted to reports on Federally funded programs on aging, legislative actions, news of state programs. Includes a conference calendar and review of recent publications.

Annual Review of Experimental Aging Research. Bar Harbor, Maine 04609. (Annually).

Issued each April, this publication on clinical and experimental research is concerned with the process of aging and the aged. Includes both human and animal research and is multidisciplinary.

Current Literature on Aging. The National Council on the Aging. 1828 L Street, N. W. Washington, D. C. 20036. (Quarterly).

Annotated references of recent books and articles pertaining to aging reported under topical headings.

Dynamic Maturity. American Association of Retired Persons. 1909 K Street, N. W. Washington, D. C. 20049. (Bi-monthly).

This is the official publication of Action for Independent Maturity (AIM), a division of the Association. Includes both informational and entertaining articles designed for its audience of persons in the middle years.

Educational Gerontology. Hemisphere Publishing Corporation. 1025 Vermont Avenue, N. W. Washington, D. C. 20005. (Quarterly).

This international quarterly is intended to promote "international articulation in the field of educational gerontology."

Experimental Aging Research. P. O. Box 85. Bar Harbor, Maine 04609. (Bi-monthly).

An international, interdisciplinary journal covering all areas of scientific human and animal inquiry dealing with the process of aging and the aged.

Geriatrics. Lancet Publications. 4015 West 65th Street. Minneapolis, Minnesota 55435. (Monthly).

Broad coverage of physiological and psychological aspects of the aging process and care of aged patients, such as chemotherapy, research, advances in geriatric medicine.

Geriatrics Digest. Medical Digest Group. 445 Central Avenue. Northfield, Illinois 60093. (Monthly).

This is primarily an abstracting service which alerts members of the American Geriatric Society to articles published on geriatrics. Also includes occasional articles and a few editorials and book reviews.

Gerontologist, The. Gerontological Society. One Dupont Circle. Washington, D. C. 20036. (Bi-monthly).

This journal publishes articles of professional and educational interest including such topics as social policy, historical analysis, theory, and research. Book reviews are included. Readers are kept abreast of new developments in gerontology.

Gerontology. S. Karger/Albert J. Phiebig, Inc. P. O. Box 352. White Plains, New York 10602. (Bi-monthly).

This is an international journal of experimental and clinical gerontology, formerly the two journals Gerontologia and Gerontologia Clinica. Includes contributions related to the aging processes and age related diseases in animals and man.

Harvest Years. Harvest Years Publishing Company. 104 East 40th Street. New York, New York 10016. (Monthly).

Practical advice for pre-retirees and retirees in such areas as budgets, hobbies, housing, medicine.

Human Development. S. Karger/Albert J. Phiebig, Inc. P. O. Box 352. White Plains, New York 10602. (Bi-monthly).

This perodical is devoted to the study of psychological changes and differences during the whole life span, primarily research of psychological variables, multidisciplinary investigations, and cross-cultural studies.

Industrial Gerontology. National Council on the Aging. 1828 L Street, N. W. Washington, D. C. 20036. (Quarterly).

This official publication of the National Institute of Industrial Gerontology, a program of the National Council, offers current papers on middle aged and older workers and the varied conditions and circumstances which affect them.

International Journal of Aging and Human Development. Baywood Publishing Company, Inc. 43 Central Drive. Farmingdale, New York 11735. (Quarterly).

An international journal of psychosocial gerontology. Formerly Aging and Human Development.

Journal of the American Geriatric Society. American Geriatric Society. 10 Columbus Circle. New York, New York 10010. (Monthly).

Emphasis is focused on the geriatric patient rather than the aged in general. Although written for the medical practitioner, it contains many articles easily understood by those outside this profession. Articles often reflect studies of medical management and institutional care.

Journal of Geriatric Psychiatry. International Universities Press. 315 Fifth Avenue. New York, New York 10016. (Semi-annual).

This official journal of the Boston Society for Gerontological Psychiatry is designed to present recent findings and new information in the field of geriatric psychiatry and to serve as a forum for the exchange of ideas. The audience is psychiatrists, psychologists, social workers, social scientists and medical personnel interested in the aged.

Journal of Gerontological Nursing. Charles B. Slack, Inc. 6900 Grove Road. Thorofare, New Jersey 08086. (Bi-monthly).

This periodical covers theory, methodology and the body of information pertaining to geriatric nursing.

Journal of Gerontology. Gerontological Society. One Dupont Circle. Washington, D. C. 20036. (Bi-monthly).

The official journal of the Society, which is devoted to research on aging. Articles pertain to: biological and medical sciences, psychology and social sciences, and social gerontology. Includes also book reviews and a current publications list.

Mature Years. United Methodist Publishing House. 201 Eighth Avenue, South. Nashville, Tennessee 37203. (Quarterly).

A religious publication directed to the old and/or retired. Considerable emphasis is placed on how the aged can serve their communities. Fiction sometimes included.

Memo. National Institute of Senior Centers. National Council on the Aging. 1828 L Street, N. W. Washington, D. C. 20036.

A monthly newsletter that provides a variety of information concerning senior centers, including Federal programs, legislation, center programs, and related topics.

Modern Maturity. American Association of Retired Persons. 1909 K Street, N. W. Washington, D. C. 20049. (Bi-monthly).

The official journal of AARP covers topics of interest to their membership, including such areas as: social welfare, education, health, political developments and entertainment.

NRTA Journal. National Retired Teachers Association. 215 Long Beach Boulevard. Long Beach, California 90802. (Bi-monthly).

This publication offers articles on all aspects of retirement from income to health for members of the Association.

Nursing Homes. Cogswell House, Inc. 222 Wisconsin Avenue. Lake Forest, Illinois 60045. (Bi-monthly).

Topics included are concerned with departmental operations and services, governmental regulations and facilities' planning. The service reach of the publication encompasses all types of long term health care and residential facilities.

Omega. Baywood Publishing Company, Inc. 43 Central Drive. Farmingdale, New York 11735. (Quarterly).

An international journal devoted to psychological studies on dying, death, grief, suicide and behavioral effects. Not limited to the aged.

Perspective on Aging. National Council on the Aging. 1828 L Street, N. W. Washington, D. C. 20036. (Bi-monthly).

This journal offers brief articles incorporating reports on activities of older persons, Federal programs, and special topics, as well as regular features, e.g., book reviews, public policy developments and summary of Council activities.

Retirement Life. National Association of Retired Civil Employees. 1909 Q Street, N. W. Washington, D. C. 20009. (Monthly).

This publication is directed toward those drawing Federal civil service employee retirement benefits. Most of the material concerns laws, legislation and programs governing annuitants and their survivors. Sometimes includes more general articles on aging.

Senate Special Committee on Aging Memorandum. United States Senate Special Sommittee on Aging. G-225 Senate Office Building. Washington, D. C. 20510. (Frequent, irregular schedule).

This bulletin supplements hearings and studies of the Committee, reports on legislation, programs, and the status of bills in Congress.

Senior Advocate. Senior Advocates International, Inc. 1825 K Street, N. W. Washington, D. C. 20006. (Bi-monthly).

This journal of Senior Advocates International, a public advocacy organization of persons over 50 years of age, gives information about the organization programs, legislative developments, and a strong emphasis on consumerism.

Senior Citizens News. National Council of Senior Citizens. 1511 K Street, N. W. Washington, D. C. 20510. (Monthly).

A bulletin which emphasizes coverage of legislation of interest to older persons nation-wide.

Social Security Bulletin. Office of Research and Statistics. Social Security Administration. Superintendent of Documents. U. S. Government Printing Office. Washington, D. C. 20402. (Monthly).

A publication of investigative study results and statistical information on Social Security. Includes reports on Federal legislation, program developments and assessments.

AUTHOR-EDITOR INDEX

A

B

C

H

L

Mc

M

N

O

P

T

U

V

W

32092

HQ
1061 Rooke
R777 Gerontology
1978